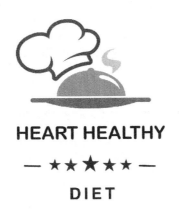

HEART HEALTHY

— ★★★★★ —

DIET

The

Heart Healthy

COOKBOOK FOR BEGINNERS

Delicious, Low-Sodium and Low-Cholesterol, Nutritious
Recipes for Lowering Blood Pressure, with Easy Diet
Habits for Optimal Health at Any Age - SCIENCE-BASED

+

42-Day Meal Plan

Dr. Jennifer M. Walker

Contents

Detailed
Table of Contents

Chapter 9: Side Dishes 68

Chapter 10: Soups 77

Chapter 11: Vegetarian Dishes 84

Appendix 1: Measurement Conversion Chart........................123

Index........................125

Introduction

Nourishing Your Heart

Welcome to a journey toward nurturing one of the most vital organs in your body—the heart. Within these pages, we'll embark on a discovery of the profound impact that our dietary choices hold over the health and well-being of this remarkable powerhouse within us.

The heart, tirelessly beating an average of 100,000 times a day, is the epicenter of our vitality. Yet, in our modern lives filled with convenience and fast-paced living, we often overlook the profound influence that what we eat wields upon its health and longevity.

In this exploration, we'll delve into the fundamental relationship between the foods we consume and the resilience of our heart. We'll uncover not just the importance of healthy eating, but the actionable steps and insightful knowledge necessary to make informed choices for a heart-nourishing diet.

Throughout history, cultures have recognized the symbolic significance of the heart—a center of life, emotions, and strength. Our journey together aims to honor this significance by equipping you with the tools to sustain and cherish your heart's health.

Prepare to unravel the mysteries of nutrition, unlock the potential of wholesome foods, and embark on a path that celebrates not just the act of eating but the profound impact it has on the beat that keeps us alive—the rhythm of our heart.

So, let us venture forth, pen in hand, eager to script a tale of wellness, vibrancy, and the harmonious relationship between the sustenance we choose and the heart that sustains us.

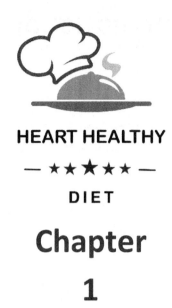

HEART HEALTHY

— ★★★★★ —

DIET

Chapter
1

The Foundation of Heart-Healthy Eating

A heart-healthy diet offers a multitude of benefits that extend beyond just cardiovascular health. Here are some key advantages:

Cardiovascular Health

1. **Heart Disease Prevention:** Reducing the risk of heart disease by managing cholesterol levels, blood pressure, and preventing arterial plaque buildup.

2. **Lower Blood Pressure:** Consuming foods rich in potassium, magnesium, and fiber helps regulate blood pressure, reducing strain on the heart.

3. **Cholesterol Management:** Promoting a balance of healthy fats and reducing intake of saturated and trans fats can lower LDL (bad) cholesterol levels and increase HDL (good) cholesterol.

Overall Health and Wellness

4. **Weight Management:** A heart-healthy diet often leads to better weight control, reducing the risk of obesity-related complications.

5. **Reduced Risk of Type 2 Diabetes:** Whole grains, fruits, and vegetables in such diets help regulate blood sugar levels, decreasing the risk of developing diabetes.

6. **Improved Digestive Health:** High fiber content in fruits, vegetables, and whole grains promotes healthy digestion and reduces the risk of digestive issues.

Long-Term Well-being

7. **Increased Longevity:** Lowering the risk of heart disease, stroke, and other cardiovascular issues contributes to a longer and healthier life.

8. **Enhanced Energy Levels:** Nutrient-dense foods provide sustained energy, reducing fatigue and promoting overall vitality.

9. **Better Mental Health:** Healthy eating habits have been linked to improved mood, cognitive function, and a reduced risk of mental health issues.

Quality of Life

10. **Enhanced Immune Function:** Nutrient-rich diets support a robust immune system, aiding in the body's defense against illnesses.

11. **Better Sleep:** A balanced diet contributes to improved sleep quality, ensuring better rest and rejuvenation.

12. **Overall Vitality:** The combined effects of a heart-healthy diet contribute to an overall sense of well-being, vitality, and a higher quality of life.

Adopting a heart-healthy diet not only supports the cardiovascular system but also significantly impacts overall health, well-being, and longevity.

Basic Principles of a Heart-Healthy Diet

1. **Balanced Macronutrients:** A heart-healthy diet emphasizes a balance of carbohydrates, lean proteins, and healthy fats. Focus on whole grains, lean proteins (such as fish, poultry, beans), and sources of healthy fats like avocados, nuts, and olive oil.

2. **Abundance of Fruits and Vegetables:** Incorporate a variety of colorful fruits and vegetables into your meals. They are rich in antioxidants, vitamins, and minerals that support heart health and reduce the risk of cardiovascular diseases.

3. **Limit Saturated and Trans Fats:** Reduce intake of saturated fats found in red meat, full-fat dairy, and processed foods. Avoid trans fats often found in fried and commercially baked goods as they can raise LDL cholesterol levels.

4. **Healthy Cooking Methods:** Opt for cooking methods that involve minimal use of oil and avoid deep-frying. Grilling, steaming, baking, or sautéing with healthier oils like olive or canola oil are better alternatives.

5. **Moderation in Salt Intake:** High sodium intake can elevate blood pressure. Aim to reduce salt intake by using herbs, spices, and other flavorings to season food instead of relying on salt.

6. **Limit Refined Sugars:** Excessive sugar consumption can contribute to weight gain and heart issues. Minimize intake of sugary beverages, processed snacks, and desserts.

7. **Portion Control:** Be mindful of portion sizes to avoid overeating, which can lead to weight gain and strain on the heart.

Why Cardiovascular Problems Occur

Cardiovascular issues often arise due to a combination of factors:

1. **Poor Diet:** Diets high in saturated fats, trans fats, sodium, and refined sugars contribute to conditions like hypertension, high cholesterol, and obesity, all of which are risk factors for heart disease.

2. **Lack of Physical Activity:** Sedentary lifestyles contribute to weight gain, high blood pressure, and other conditions that strain the cardiovascular system.

3. **Smoking and Excessive Alcohol Consumption:** These habits increase the risk of heart disease by damaging blood vessels, raising blood pressure, and elevating the risk of blood clots.

4. **Genetic Factors:** Family history of heart disease or genetic predispositions can increase the likelihood of cardiovascular issues.

5. **Chronic Stress:** Long-term stress can contribute to high blood pressure and heart problems.

6. **Medical Conditions:** Conditions like diabetes, obesity, and metabolic syndrome can significantly increase the risk of heart disease.

Understanding these principles and the factors contributing to cardiovascular issues can empower individuals to make informed choices and take proactive steps toward a heart-healthy lifestyle.

What cardiovascular problems can lead to

Cardiovascular problems yield profound consequences, dramatically affecting health. Heart attacks, stemming from reduced blood flow to the heart, can cause irreversible damage, while strokes, triggered by blood clots in the brain, result in neurological impairments. Long-term issues often culminate in heart failure, manifesting as fatigue and fluid retention. Aneurysms and peripheral artery disease bring risks of life-threatening complications and impaired mobility. Chronic cardiovascular problems may lead to kidney damage, elevating the risk of kidney failure. Beyond physical repercussions, arrhythmias and hypertension contribute to palpitations and arterial strain. Emotional tolls include heightened stress and anxiety. These cumulative effects markedly diminish the quality of life, underscoring the importance of proactive measures such as regular check-ups, lifestyle adjustments, and consistent medical management to mitigate these potentially severe consequences.

Macro and micronutrients

In our quest for a resilient heart, understanding the cornerstone principles of a nourishing diet lays the groundwork for a robust and enduring relationship with our cardiovascular health.

Exploring Macronutrients

At the heart of every meal lie the three essential macronutrients: carbohydrates, proteins, and fats. Each plays a pivotal role in sustaining our body's functions, but their quality and balance hold the key to nurturing our heart. Carbohydrates provide energy, proteins aid in repair and growth, while fats serve as vital building blocks and sources of essential nutrients.

The Role of Micronutrients and Antioxidants

Beyond these macronutrients, micronutrients—vitamins, minerals, and antioxidants—paint a more intricate canvas of health. They act as guardians, fortifying our heart against oxidative stress and bolstering its resilience. Understanding their significance in maintaining a well-functioning cardiovascular system is pivotal to crafting a diet that thrives on these nutritional powerhouses.

Choosing Quality Foods

The landscape of modern nutrition is often cluttered with choices, yet discerning the nutritious from the detrimental is a vital skill. Selecting whole, unprocessed foods over their refined counterparts is a cornerstone of a heart-healthy diet. It's not just about what we eat but the quality of the ingredients that nourish us.

In this chapter, we lay the groundwork for our journey toward a heart-conscious diet. By unraveling the significance of macronutrients, delving into the realm of micronutrients, and learning to distinguish between beneficial and harmful food choices, we set the stage for a diet that resonates with the rhythm of a healthy heart.

This chapter aims to introduce readers to the fundamental components of a heart-healthy diet, emphasizing the importance of macronutrients, micronutrients, and the quality of food choices in nurturing cardiovascular health. Adjust or expand upon these ideas to suit the specific focus or tone of your book!

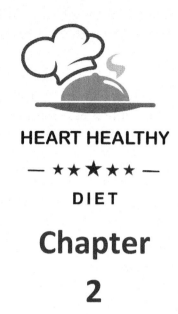

HEART HEALTHY

— ★★★★★ —

DIET

Chapter 2

Recommendations and Restrictions on Foods

Food that is permissible to consume

A heart-healthy diet emphasizes nutrient-rich, whole foods that support cardiovascular health. Here are examples of foods typically recommended:

Fruits

Berries

- **Blueberries:** Rich in antioxidants, vitamins C and K, and fiber.
- **Strawberries:** High in antioxidants and vitamin C, known for their heart-protective benefits.
- **Raspberries:** Packed with fiber, antioxidants, and various vitamins.

Citrus Fruits

- **Oranges:** High in vitamin C, potassium, and fiber, known to support heart health.
- **Grapefruits:** Rich in antioxidants and fiber, known to help lower cholesterol.
- **Lemons:** High in vitamin C and antioxidants, beneficial for heart health.

Other Heart-Healthy Fruits

- **Apples:** High in soluble fiber and antioxidants.
- **Pears:** Rich in fiber and vitamin C, promoting heart health.
- **Bananas:** Good source of potassium and vitamins C and B6, beneficial for heart function.
- **Mangoes:** High in vitamins A and C, as well as fiber and antioxidants.
- **Papayas:** Rich in vitamins C and A, antioxidants, and fiber.

- **Grapes:** Contain antioxidants like resveratrol, promoting heart health.
- **Kiwi:** High in vitamin C, fiber, and antioxidants.
- **Watermelon:** Contains antioxidants like lycopene, supporting heart health.
- **Cherries:** Rich in antioxidants, fiber, and potassium.

Dried Fruits (In Moderation)

- **Raisins:** Contain fiber, potassium, and antioxidants.
- **Dried Apricots:** High in fiber, vitamins A and C, and potassium.

Vegetables

Leafy Greens

- **Spinach:** Rich in vitamins A, C, and K, as well as iron and antioxidants.
- **Kale:** High in vitamins A, C, and K, and a good source of fiber and antioxidants.
- **Swiss Chard:** Packed with vitamins A, K, and C, as well as magnesium and potassium.
- **Collard Greens:** Rich in vitamins A, C, and K, and a good source of calcium and fiber.

Cruciferous Vegetables

- **Broccoli:** High in vitamins C, K, and folate, as well as antioxidants.
- **Cauliflower:** Rich in vitamins C and K, and a good source of fiber and antioxidants.
- **Brussels Sprouts:** High in vitamins C and K, fiber, and antioxidants.
- **Cabbage:** Contains vitamins C and K, and provides antioxidants.

Colorful Vegetables

- **Bell Peppers:** High in vitamins C and A, and a good source of antioxidants.
- **Carrots:** Rich in beta-carotene, vitamins A and K, and fiber.
- **Tomatoes:** Contain vitamins C and K, as well as lycopene, a heart-protective antioxidant.
- **Beets:** High in vitamins C and B9, fiber, and antioxidants.

Root Vegetables

- **Sweet Potatoes:** Rich in vitamins A and C, fiber, and antioxidants.
- **Potatoes (with skin):** Good source of potassium, vitamin C, and fiber.

Other Heart-Healthy Vegetables

- **Asparagus:** High in vitamins K and folate, and a good source of fiber.
- **Zucchini:** Contains vitamins C and B6, and is low in calories.
- **Eggplant:** Rich in fiber and antioxidants, and low in calories.
- **Green Beans:** Good source of vitamins C and K, and a moderate source of fiber.

Whole Grains

Wheat-Based Grains

- **Whole Wheat:** Contains all parts of the wheat kernel, providing fiber, vitamins, and minerals.
- **Whole Wheat Bread:** Made from whole wheat flour, a good source of fiber and nutrients.

- **Whole Wheat Pasta:** High in fiber and nutrients compared to refined pasta.

Other Grains

- **Oats:** Rich in soluble fiber, known to help lower cholesterol levels.
- **Brown Rice:** Contains more nutrients and fiber compared to white rice.
- **Quinoa:** High in protein, fiber, and various vitamins and minerals.
- **Barley:** Packed with fiber, vitamins, and antioxidants.
- **Bulgur:** High in fiber and a good source of vitamins and minerals.
- **Farro:** Contains fiber, protein, and various nutrients.
- **Millet:** Rich in nutrients and a good source of fiber.
- **Whole Grain Corn:** Provides fiber, vitamins, and minerals.
- **Amaranth:** High in protein, fiber, and various nutrients.
- **Buckwheat:** Rich in antioxidants and fiber.
- **Rye:** Contains fiber, vitamins, and minerals.

Lean Proteins

Poultry

- **Skinless Chicken Breast:** High in protein and low in saturated fat.
- **Skinless Turkey Breast:** Lean source of protein, vitamins, and minerals.
- **Ground Turkey (Lean):** Choose lean ground turkey for lower fat content.

Fish

- **Salmon:** Rich in omega-3 fatty acids, protein, and nutrients beneficial for heart health.
- **Mackerel:** High in omega-3s and a good source of protein.
- **Trout:** Contains omega-3s and is a lean protein option.
- **Sardines:** Packed with omega-3s and protein.

Shellfish

- **Shrimp:** Low in calories and saturated fat, a good source of protein.
- **Scallops:** High in protein and low in fat.
- **Crab:** Lean source of protein and various nutrients.

Lean Meats (in Moderation)

- **Lean Cuts of Beef:** Look for cuts like sirloin or tenderloin, trimmed of visible fat.
- **Pork Tenderloin:** Lean and a good source of protein.
- **Veal:** Lean meat option if consumed in moderation.

Plant-Based Proteins

- **Tofu:** Soy-based protein with low saturated fat content.
- **Tempeh:** Fermented soy protein, a good source of protein and nutrients.
- **Edamame:** Young soybeans, low in fat and a good source of protein.
- **Lentils:** High in protein and fiber, low in fat.

Healthy Fats

Plant-Based Oils

- **Olive Oil:** Rich in monounsaturated fats and antioxidants, beneficial for heart health.
- **Avocado Oil**: Contains monounsaturated fats and antioxidants, suitable for cooking.
- **Canola Oil**: High in monounsaturated fats and omega-3s, good for cooking.

Nuts and Seeds

- **Almonds:** High in monounsaturated fats, fiber, and antioxidants.
- **Walnuts:** Rich in omega-3 fatty acids, beneficial for heart health.
- **Pistachios:** Contain healthy fats, fiber, and antioxidants.
- **Chia Seeds:** High in omega-3s, fiber, and protein.
- **Flaxseeds:** Rich in omega-3s, fiber, and lignans (antioxidants).

Fatty Fish

- **Salmon:** Abundant in omega-3 fatty acids, beneficial for heart health.
- **Mackerel:** Rich in omega-3s and a good source of healthy fats.
- **Sardines:** Packed with omega-3s and nutrients beneficial for heart health.

Dairy and Alternatives

- **Low-Fat Dairy:** Milk, yogurt, cheese—sources of calcium and protein.
- **Plant-Based Milk:** Almond, soy, oat milk—lower in saturated fats.

Herbs, Spices, and Flavorings

- **Herbs:** Basil, parsley, cilantro—add flavor without sodium.
- **Spices:** Turmeric, cinnamon, ginger—have antioxidant properties.

Other

- **Dark Chocolate:** High cocoa content with antioxidants in moderation.
- **Green Tea:** Contains antioxidants linked to heart health.

A heart-healthy diet focuses on whole, minimally processed foods rich in nutrients while limiting foods high in unhealthy fats, added sugars, and excessive sodium. It's about creating a balanced and varied diet to support cardiovascular health.

Foods to Limit or Avoid

foods that are generally discouraged or limited in a heart-healthy diet due to their high saturated fats, trans fats, sodium content, or added sugars:

Foods High in Saturated and Trans Fats

- **Fried Foods:** French fries, fried chicken, etc., high in unhealthy fats.
- **Processed Meats:** Sausages, bacon, hot dogs, and certain deli meats.
- **High-Fat Dairy:** Full-fat cheese, cream, and certain high-fat yogurts.
- **Commercially Baked Goods:** Pastries, cookies, and cakes often made with trans fats.

Excessive Sodium Foods

- **Canned Soups:** Often high in sodium content.
- **Processed Meats:** Cured meats and certain cold cuts.
- **Fast Food:** Burgers, fries, and other fast-food items are often high in sodium.

Refined Carbohydrates and Sugary Foods

- **White Bread:** Lacks fiber and nutrients found in whole grains.
- **Sugary Snacks:** Candies, sugary cereals, and sweetened beverages.
- **Baked Goods:** Pastries, cakes, and desserts with added sugars.

High Sodium Condiments

- **Soy Sauce:** High in sodium, contributing to increased blood pressure.
- **Store-Bought Salad Dressings:** Many contain high amounts of added salt.

Minimizing or avoiding these foods helps lower the intake of unhealthy fats, excessive sodium, and added sugars, which can contribute to heart disease, high blood pressure, and other cardiovascular issues.

Spices and herbs that can partially replace salt

Herbs

- **Basil** – great for vegetable dishes, pasta, and sauces.
- **Oregano** – pairs well with tomato dishes, fish, and meat.
- **Thyme** – adds depth to soups, casseroles, and chicken.
- **Rosemary** – perfect for potatoes, fish, and meats.
- **Dill** – enhances the flavor of fish, potatoes, and salads.

Spices

- **Garlic (fresh or powder)** – adds rich flavor to soups, vegetables, and meats.
- **Onion (powder or fresh)** – boosts the taste of most dishes.
- **Turmeric** – adds a warm flavor and a beautiful color.
- **Ginger** – works well with vegetables, meat, and tea.
- **Paprika (regular or smoked)** – gives dishes a rich taste.
- Black pepper and cayenne pepper – add a spicy kick.

Other Flavor Enhancers

- **Lemon juice or zest** – enhances the taste of fish, chicken, and salads.
- **Apple cider vinegar** – improves the flavor of vegetables and soups.
- **Nutritional yeast** – adds a cheesy flavor without salt.

These natural substitutes will help make your meals flavorful and heart-friendly.

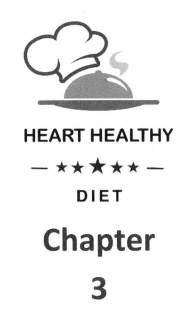

HEART HEALTHY

— ★★★★★ —

DIET

Chapter
3

Physical activity and a positive attitude

Physical Activity

Improved Heart Strength and Efficiency

Regular physical activity, especially aerobic exercises like brisk walking, running, or cycling, strengthens the heart muscle. This enhanced strength allows the heart to pump blood more efficiently, improving circulation and reducing strain on the cardiovascular system.

Lowered Blood Pressure

Consistent exercise can help manage and reduce high blood pressure, a significant risk factor for heart disease. It helps keep the arteries and blood vessels more elastic, allowing blood to flow more freely and maintaining healthy blood pressure levels.

Healthy Cholesterol Levels

Physical activity increases high-density lipoprotein (HDL) cholesterol—the "good" cholesterol—while lowering levels of low-density lipoprotein (LDL) cholesterol—the "bad" cholesterol. This balance supports better heart health by preventing the buildup of plaque in the arteries.

Better Weight Management

Regular exercise contributes to weight management and weight loss, reducing the risk of obesity, which is linked to various cardiovascular issues. Maintaining a healthy weight through exercise can significantly lower the risk of heart disease and related conditions.

Enhanced Circulation and Oxygenation

Exercise boosts blood circulation, improving the flow of oxygen-rich blood throughout the body, including the heart. This supports the health of the heart and other organs, improving overall vitality and reducing the workload on the heart.

Reduced Stress and Inflammation
Physical activity triggers the release of endorphins, promoting a sense of well-being and reducing stress. Additionally, it helps control inflammation in the body, which can contribute to heart disease and other chronic conditions.

Improved Heart Rate and Rhythm
Regular exercise helps regulate and maintain a healthy heart rate and rhythm. It strengthens the heart's electrical system, reducing the risk of irregular heartbeats and other heart-related issues.

Long-Term Heart Health
Engaging in regular physical activity significantly lowers the risk of developing various cardiovascular diseases, including coronary artery disease, heart attacks, and strokes. It contributes to a longer, healthier life by supporting overall heart health.

Incorporating various forms of exercise into your routine, following recommended guidelines, and maintaining consistency can significantly benefit your cardiovascular system and contribute to a healthier heart.

Exercising regularly is an integral part of a heart-healthy lifestyle. Here are some exercises suitable for promoting cardiovascular health:

Aerobic/Cardio Exercises
- **Brisk Walking:** An accessible and effective way to boost heart health.
- **Running or Jogging:** Helps improve cardiovascular endurance.
- **Cycling:** Low-impact and beneficial for heart health.
- **Swimming:** Engages multiple muscle groups and is gentle on joints.
- **Dancing:** Fun and effective for cardiovascular fitness.
- **Rowing:** Great for upper and lower body workout while engaging the heart.
- **Jump Rope:** Increases heart rate and improves coordination.

Interval Training
- **High-Intensity Interval Training (HIIT):** Alternating between bursts of intense activity and rest periods, great for cardiovascular health.

Strength Training
- **Bodyweight Exercises:** Push-ups, squats, lunges, and planks can all contribute to muscle strength.

Flexibility and Balance
- **Yoga:** Enhances flexibility, balance, and can help reduce stress.
- **Pilates:** Improves core strength and stability.
- **Tai Chi:** Gentle movements that promote balance and relaxation.

Tips:
- **Consult a Professional:** Before starting a new exercise routine, especially if you have underlying health conditions, consult a healthcare professional or a certified fitness trainer.
- **Consistency is Key:** Aim for at least 150 minutes of moderate-intensity exercise per week or 75 minutes of vigorous-intensity exercise, along with strength training exercises at least two days per week.

Combining different types of exercises that you enjoy can make it easier to stick to a routine. The key is to find activities that you find enjoyable and sustainable to maintain a regular exercise regimen that supports your heart health.

Positive Attitude

Maintaining a positive mental attitude is a powerful asset in the battle against cardiovascular diseases. Here's why it matters:

Stress Management

A positive mental attitude can aid in managing stress, which is a significant contributor to heart disease. Stress increases blood pressure, strains the cardiovascular system, and contributes to unhealthy coping behaviors like overeating or smoking. Adopting a positive outlook can help mitigate stress and its impact on heart health.

Healthy Habits Adherence

A positive mindset often aligns with healthier lifestyle choices. People with an optimistic outlook are more likely to adhere to heart-healthy habits like regular exercise, maintaining a balanced diet, and avoiding harmful behaviors like smoking or excessive alcohol consumption.

Resilience Against Adversity

A positive mental attitude fosters resilience when facing challenges, including health-related setbacks. It enables individuals to cope better with the complexities of managing a cardiovascular condition, encouraging perseverance, and fostering a proactive approach to recovery.

Improved Overall Well-being

Positivity and optimism contribute to overall well-being, promoting emotional resilience, and reducing the risk of depression or anxiety, which can have adverse effects on heart health. A happier outlook can lead to a healthier heart.

Better Adherence to Treatment

Individuals with a positive mindset are often more proactive and consistent in following their treatment plans. Whether it's medication adherence, attending medical appointments, or engaging in rehabilitation programs, a positive attitude can boost commitment to recovery.

Social Support and Connection

A positive mental attitude encourages seeking and nurturing social connections. Strong social support has been linked to better heart health outcomes, as it provides emotional support, reduces isolation, and offers encouragement in managing cardiovascular conditions.

Mind-Body Connection

Recognizing the mind-body connection is crucial. A positive mental attitude complements physical efforts in managing heart health. Meditation, mindfulness, and relaxation techniques can aid in reducing stress, promoting calmness, and supporting heart health.

Long-Term Resilience

Maintaining a positive outlook contributes to long-term resilience in coping with the challenges associated with cardiovascular diseases. It fosters hope, motivation, and the determination to lead a fulfilling life despite the condition.

A positive mental attitude isn't a cure, but it's a powerful complement to medical treatment and a healthy lifestyle in the fight against cardiovascular diseases. Cultivating positivity, managing stress, and embracing optimism can significantly contribute to better heart health outcomes and overall well-being. Believe in yourself and take action, and you will succeed!

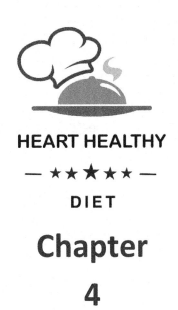

HEART HEALTHY

— ★ ★ ★ ★ ★ —

DIET

Chapter

4

42-Day Meal Plan

Discover the path to a healthier heart with our comprehensive 42-day meal plan, meticulously crafted to support cardiovascular wellness. This heart-healthy meal plan emphasizes the importance of nutrient-dense foods, featuring an array of fruits, vegetables, whole grains, lean proteins, and healthy fats. Each day offers a balanced combination of breakfast, lunch, dinner, and snacks, ensuring you receive essential vitamins, minerals, and antioxidants to promote heart health. Our recipes are designed to be delicious and easy to prepare, making it simple to incorporate heart-friendly foods into your daily routine. From flavorful salads and hearty soups to satisfying main courses and wholesome snacks, this meal plan provides a variety of options to keep your taste buds excited and your heart strong. Take the first step towards a healthier you with our 42-day meal plan and enjoy the benefits of eating well for your heart.

WEEK 1					
	Breakfast	**Lunch**	**Dinner**	**Snack**	**Dessert**
Day 1	Almond Milk Oatmeal with Sliced Bananas	Stuffed Portobello Mushrooms with Quinoa and Spinach	Pan-Seared Trout with Almond Butter, Stir-Fried Snow Peas and Red Peppers	Spiced Chickpea Crunchies	Avocado Chocolate Mousse
Day 2	Quinoa Breakfast Bowl with Fresh Fruits	Mediterranean Chickpea and Lemon Soup	Skinless Turkey Meatballs in Marinara, Tomato, Basil, and Mozzarella Caprese	Crispy Kale Chips with Sea Salt	Matcha and Almond Cookies

	Breakfast	Lunch	Dinner	Snack	Dessert
Day 3	Steel-Cut Oats with Apple and Cinnamon	Sesame-Crusted Chicken with Steamed Vegetables	Zesty Lime and Cilantro Cauliflower Rice, Lemon-Herb Grilled Salmon	Roasted Sweet Potato Rounds	Vegan Lemon Sorbet
Day 4	Quinoa Breakfast Bowl with Fresh Fruits	Saffron-Infused Seafood Paella	Creamy Avocado Pesto Zoodles, Thai-Style Beef Salad	Chia Seed and Berry Yogurt Parfait	Strawberry and Basil Frozen Yogurt
Day 5	Baked Avocado Eggs with Fresh Salsa	Mediterranean Chickpea and Lemon Soup	Buffalo Chicken Stuffed Sweet Potatoes, Broccoli and Cranberry Coleslaw	Olive and Walnut Tapenade on Whole-Grain Toast	Coconut and Berry Chia Pudding
Day 6	Low-Fat Greek Yogurt Parfait	Sesame-Crusted Ahi Tuna Steaks, Spicy Thai Mango and Tofu Salad	Lemon-Herb Grilled Salmon, Sautéed Spinach with Garlic and Lemon	Almond and Cranberry Trail Mix	Matcha and Almond Cookies
Day 7	Avocado Toast with Poached Egg	Thai-Style Beef Salad, Grilled Corn with Chili-Lime Butter	Stir-Fried Tofu with Sesame and Broccoli	Roasted Sweet Potato Rounds	Maple-Roasted Peaches

WEEK 2

	Breakfast	Lunch	Dinner	Snack	Dessert
Day 1	Whole-Grain Pancakes with Sugar-Free Maple Syrup	Buffalo Chicken Stuffed Sweet Potatoes	Red Lentil Dahl with Brown Rice, Spicy Shrimp Ceviche	Veggie Hummus Dip Cups	Gluten-Free Carrot Cake with Cashew Frosting
Day 2	Sweet Potato Hash with Black Beans	Sesame-Crusted Ahi Tuna Steaks, Tomato, Basil, and Mozzarella Caprese	Vegetarian Taco Salad with Black Beans, Jerk-Spiced Turkey Breast	Veggie Hummus Dip Cups	Dark Chocolate and Almond Bark
Day 3	Cauliflower Rice Breakfast Stir-Fry	Sous-Vide Pork Loin with Cherry Sauce, Avocado and Pomegranate Seed Salad	Vegetable and Lentil Shepherd's Pie	Sundried Tomato and Basil Pinwheels	Cinnamon-Spiced Baked Apples
Day 4	Tofu Benedict with Avocado Sauce	Lemon-Herb Grilled Salmon, Spicy Thai Mango and Tofu Salad	Stir-Fried Tofu with Sesame and Broccoli	Zucchini Pizza Bites	Banana and Walnut Bread

Day 5	Veggie-Loaded Breakfast Casserole	Curried Cauliflower and Carrot Soup	Balsamic Glazed Pork Tenderloin, Avocado and Pomegranate Seed Salad	Almond and Cranberry Trail Mix	Vegan Lemon Sorbet
Day 6	Baked Avocado Eggs with Fresh Salsa	Jerk-Spiced Turkey Breast, Avocado and Pomegranate Seed Salad	Grilled Eggplant and Zucchini Lasagna	Apple Slices with Almond Butter Drizzle	Maple-Roasted Peaches
Day 7	Smoked Salmon and Cucumber Bagel (Whole Grain)	Sesame-Crusted Chicken with Steamed Vegetables	Lemon and Herb Couscous, Garlic and Rosemary Sea Bass	Spiced Chickpea Crunchies	Gluten-Free Carrot Cake with Cashew Frosting

WEEK 3

	Breakfast	Lunch	Dinner	Snack	Dessert
Day 1	Baked Avocado Eggs with Fresh Salsa	Cumin-Spiced Carrot and Parsnip Fries, Broccoli and Cranberry Coleslaw	Herbed Roast Beef with Root Vegetables, Balsamic-Glazed Brussels Sprouts	Apple Slices with Almond Butter Drizzle	Maple-Roasted Peaches
Day 2	Sweet Potato Hash with Black Beans	Sweet Corn and Bell Pepper Chowder	Pan-Seared Trout with Almond Butter, Smoky Paprika Roasted Potatoes	Veggie Hummus Dip Cups	Raspberry Almond Tartlets
Day 3	Nut Butter and Banana Breakfast Sandwich	Garlic and Rosemary Sweet Potato Wedges, Avocado and Pomegranate Seed Salad	Balsamic Chicken and Mushroom Skillet	Zucchini Pizza Bites	Avocado Chocolate Mousse
Day 4	Tofu Benedict with Avocado Sauce	Lobster Salad with Baby Greens, Parmesan Zucchini Noodles	Zesty Lime and Cilantro Cauliflower Rice, Green Apple and Walnut Crunch Salad	Roasted Sweet Potato Rounds	Cinnamon-Spiced Baked Apples
Day 5	Zucchini Bread Overnight Oats	Lean Beef Stir-Fry with Broccoli and Peppers	Thai Vegetable Curry with Coconut Milk, Tomato, Basil, and Mozzarella Caprese	Zucchini Pizza Bites	Coconut and Berry Chia Pudding

| Day 6 | Chickpea Scramble Tofu Wrap | Honey-Mustard Glazed Salmon, Curried Lentil and Mixed Greens Salad | Grilled Eggplant and Zucchini Lasagna | Chia Seed and Berry Yogurt Parfait | Strawberry and Basil Frozen Yogurt |
| Day 7 | Low-Fat Greek Yogurt Parfait | Spiced Pumpkin and Butternut Squash Soup | Apple-Glazed Pork Loin, Spinach and Strawberry Summer Salad | Zucchini Pizza Bites | Cinnamon-Spiced Baked Apples |

WEEK 4					
	Breakfast	**Lunch**	**Dinner**	**Snack**	**Dessert**
Day 1	Veggie-Loaded Breakfast Casserole	Asian-Style Lettuce Wraps with Ground Chicken	Cumin-Spiced Carrot and Parsnip Fries, Broccoli and Cranberry Coleslaw	Sundried Tomato and Basil Pinwheels	Banana and Walnut Bread
Day 2	Kale and Turkey Sausage Breakfast Burrito	Veal Scallopini with Lemon and Capers, Mediterranean Farro Salad with Lemon-Tahini Dressing	Slow-Cooked Turkey Chili	Olive and Walnut Tapenade on Whole-Grain Toast	Raspberry Almond Tartlets
Day 3	Smoked Salmon and Cucumber Bagel (Whole Grain)	Beet and Ginger Detox Soup	Honey-Mustard Glazed Salmon, Kale and Quinoa Superfood Salad	Veggie Hummus Dip Cups	No-Bake Peanut Butter Energy Bites
Day 4	Shakshuka with Spinach and Chickpeas	Lemon-Dill Roasted Chicken, Shaved Brussels Sprouts and Parmesan Salad	Grilled Corn with Chili-Lime Butter	Chia Seed and Berry Yogurt Parfait	Dark Chocolate and Almond Bark
Day 5	Low-Fat Greek Yogurt Parfait	Low-Sodium Chicken Noodle Soup	Balsamic Chicken and Mushroom Skillet	Crispy Kale Chips with Sea Salt	Blueberry Oatmeal Crumble Bars
Day 6	Avocado Toast with Poached Egg	Grilled Swordfish with Pineapple Salsa, Tomato Basil and Mozzarella Caprese	Parmesan Zucchini Noodles, Jerk-Spiced Turkey Breast	Almond and Cranberry Trail Mix	No-Bake Peanut Butter Energy Bites

| Day 7 | Cauliflower Rice Breakfast Stir-Fry | Skinless Turkey Meatballs in Marinara, Mediterranean Farro Salad with Lemon-Tahini Dressing | Stir-Fried Tofu with Sesame and Broccoli | Roasted Sweet Potato Rounds | Gluten-Free Carrot Cake with Cashew Frosting |

WEEK 5

	Breakfast	Lunch	Dinner	Snack	Dessert
Day 1	Zucchini Bread Overnight Oats	Sweet Corn and Bell Pepper Chowder	Spiced Tilapia Tacos with Avocado Crema, Arugula, Orange, and Fennel Salad	Spiced Chickpea Crunchies	Raspberry Almond Tartlets
Day 2	Nut Butter and Banana Breakfast Sandwich	Balsamic Glazed Pork Tenderloin, Broccoli and Cranberry Coleslaw	Grilled Eggplant and Zucchini Lasagna	Sundried Tomato and Basil Pinwheels	Strawberry and Basil Frozen Yogurt
Day 3	Veggie-Loaded Breakfast Casserole	Sweet Corn and Bell Pepper Chowder	Garlic and Rosemary Sea Bass, Zesty Lime and Cilantro Cauliflower Rice	Chia Seed and Berry Yogurt Parfait	Banana and Walnut Bread
Day 4	Baked Avocado Eggs with Fresh Salsa	Balsamic Glazed Tofu with Roasted Vegetables	Skillet Chicken Fajitas with Whole Wheat Tortillas	Almond and Cranberry Trail Mix	Gluten-Free Carrot Cake with Cashew Frosting
Day 5	Cauliflower Rice Breakfast Stir-Fry	Spiced Tilapia Tacos with Avocado Crema	Baked Cod with Mediterranean Salsa, Broccoli and Cranberry Coleslaw	Roasted Sweet Potato Rounds	Coconut and Berry Chia Pudding
Day 6	Avocado Toast with Poached Egg	Walnut-Crusted Flounder with Spinach, Tomato, Basil, and Mozzarella Caprese	Grilled Lemon-Herb Chicken Thighs, Arugula, Orange, and Fennel Salad	Apple Slices with Almond Butter Drizzle	Maple-Roasted Peaches
Day 7	Almond Milk Oatmeal with Sliced Bananas	Vegetable Minestrone with Whole-Grain Pasta	Asian-Style Lettuce Wraps with Ground Chicken	Veggie Hummus Dip Cups	No-Bake Peanut Butter Energy Bites

WEEK 6

	Breakfast	Lunch	Dinner	Snack	Dessert
Day 1	Quinoa Breakfast Bowl with Fresh Fruits	Walnut-Crusted Flounder with Spinach, Green Apple and Walnut Crunch Salad	Tandoori Chicken with Cilantro-Mint Chutney, Smoky Paprika Roasted Potatoes	Sundried Tomato and Basil Pinwheels	Coconut and Berry Chia Pudding
Day 2	Veggie-Loaded Breakfast Casserole	Mediterranean Chickpea and Lemon Soup	Lemon-Herb Grilled Salmon, Avocado and Pomegranate Seed Salad	Baked Parmesan Zucchini Fries	Matcha and Almond Cookies
Day 3	Almond Milk Oatmeal with Sliced Bananas	Skillet Chicken Fajitas with Whole Wheat Tortillas	Quinoa Pilaf with Sun-Dried Tomatoes and Olives	Baked Parmesan Zucchini Fries	Blueberry Oatmeal Crumble Bars
Day 4	Whole-Grain Pancakes with Sugar-Free Maple Syrup	Cumin-Spiced Carrot and Parsnip Fries, Green Apple and Walnut Crunch Salad	Balsamic Chicken and Mushroom Skillet	Roasted Sweet Potato Rounds	No-Bake Peanut Butter Energy Bites
Day 5	Chickpea Scramble Tofu Wrap	Lemon-Herb Grilled Salmon, Spinach and Strawberry Summer Salad	Slow-Cooked Turkey Chili, Low-Sodium Chicken Noodle Soup	Zucchini Pizza Bites	Banana and Walnut Bread
Day 6	Avocado Toast with Poached Egg	Sesame-Crusted Ahi Tuna Steaks, Avocado and Pomegranate Seed Salad	Balsamic Glazed Tofu with Roasted Vegetables, Kale and Quinoa Superfood Salad	Olive and Walnut Tapenade on Whole-Grain Toast	Vegan Lemon Sorbet
Day 7	Smoked Salmon and Cucumber Bagel (Whole Grain)	Roasted Tomato and Basil Soup	Lemon-Herb Grilled Salmon, Green Apple and Walnut Crunch Salad	Chia Seed and Berry Yogurt Parfait	Banana and Walnut Bread

HEART HEALTHY

— ★★★★★ —

DIET

Chapter

5

Breakfast

Almond Milk Oatmeal with Sliced Bananas

Yield: 2 servings | **Prep time:** 5 minutes | **Cook time:** 10 minutes

- **1 cup old-fashioned oats**
- **2 cups unsweetened almond milk**
- **1 ripe banana, sliced**
- **1 tablespoon chia seeds**
- **1/2 teaspoon cinnamon**
- **1 tablespoon maple syrup or honey (optional)**
- **Pinch of salt**

Nutritional Information:
Approximately 270 calories,   *7g protein,*
49g carbohydrates,   *7g fat,*
9g fiber,
0mg cholesterol,
180mg sodium,
400mg potassium.

1. In a medium saucepan, bring the almond milk to a low boil over medium heat. Add a pinch of salt.
2. Stir in the old-fashioned oats and reduce heat to low. Cook for 8-10 minutes, stirring occasionally, until the oats are tender and most of the liquid has been absorbed.
3. Remove the saucepan from heat and stir in chia seeds, cinnamon, and optional maple syrup or honey.
4. Divide the oatmeal into two bowls and top each with sliced bananas.

This heart-healthy Almond Milk Oatmeal with Sliced Bananas is a perfect start to your day. Made with unsweetened almond milk, it's low in calories and free from cholesterol. The old-fashioned oats provide soluble fiber, helping to lower LDL cholesterol, while chia seeds add omega-3 fatty acids for heart protection. Cinnamon offers anti-inflammatory benefits, and bananas contribute potassium, crucial for maintaining healthy blood pressure. This warm, satisfying breakfast is both nutritious and delicious, supporting a heart-friendly diet effortlessly.

Overnight Chia Pudding with Fresh Berries

Yield: 4 servings | **Prep time:** 10 minutes | **Cook time:** 0 minutes (overnight refrigeration)

- 1/4 cup chia seeds
- 1 cup unsweetened almond milk
- 1 tablespoon maple syrup or honey (optional)
- 1 teaspoon vanilla extract
- 1/2 cup mixed fresh berries (e.g., strawberries, blueberries, raspberries)
- A pinch of salt

Nutritional Information:
Approximately 90 calories,
12g carbohydrates,   *3g protein,*
0mg cholesterol,   *4g fat,*
90mg sodium,   *5g fiber,*
120mg potassium.

5. In a medium-sized mixing bowl, combine the chia seeds, unsweetened almond milk, maple syrup or honey (if using), vanilla extract, and a pinch of salt. Stir well to ensure that all chia seeds are immersed in the liquid.
6. Cover the bowl with plastic wrap or a lid, and refrigerate overnight or at least for 6 hours.
7. Once the chia pudding has thickened, give it a good stir to break up any clumps.
8. Divide the pudding into 4 servings, and top each with an assortment of fresh berries before serving.

Overnight Chia Pudding with Fresh Berries offers a heart-healthy treat packed with omega-3 fatty acids from chia seeds and antioxidants from fresh berries. This recipe is low in cholesterol and sodium, making it ideal for a heart-healthy diet. The unsweetened almond milk provides a creamy base without added saturated fats, while optional sweeteners like maple syrup or honey add a touch of natural sweetness. Enjoy this nutrient-dense pudding as a satisfying breakfast or wholesome dessert that supports cardiovascular wellness.

Avocado Toast with Poached Egg

Yield: 2 servings | **Prep time:** 10 minutes | **Cook time:** 5 minutes

- 2 slices of whole-grain bread
- 1 ripe avocado
- 1 teaspoon lemon juice
- Salt and pepper to taste
- 2 large eggs
- 1 teaspoon white vinegar
- Optional: Red pepper flakes, for garnish
- Optional: Fresh herbs (such as parsley or chives), for garnish

Nutritional Information:
Approximately 260 calories,
26g carbohydrates,   *11g protein,*
186mg cholesterol,   *14g fat,*
280mg sodium,   *9g fiber,*
450mg potassium.

1. Toast the whole-grain bread slices to your liking.
2. While the bread is toasting, mash the ripe avocado in a bowl and mix in lemon juice, salt, and pepper.
3. Fill a medium-sized saucepan with water, add white vinegar, and bring it to a gentle simmer. Crack each egg into a small bowl, and carefully slide them into the simmering water. Poach for 3-4 minutes, or until the whites are firm but yolks are still runny.
4. Spread the mashed avocado evenly on each slice of toasted bread. Place a poached egg on top of each.
5. Season with additional salt and pepper, and if desired, garnish with red pepper flakes and fresh herbs.

This heart-healthy recipe combines the creamy goodness of avocado with the protein-packed poached egg on fiber-rich whole-grain toast. Avocados are rich in monounsaturated fats that help lower bad cholesterol levels, while whole grains support cardiovascular health by providing essential nutrients and fiber. The addition of lemon juice adds a fresh zing and helps with nutrient absorption. This quick and nutritious dish is perfect for a balanced breakfast or light lunch, supporting a heart-friendly diet.

Vegan Green Smoothie Bowl

Yield: 2 servings | **Prep time:** 10 minutes | **Cook time:** 0 minutes

- **2 cups baby spinach**
- **1 ripe banana, frozen**
- **1/2 avocado**
- **1 cup unsweetened almond milk**
- **1 tablespoon chia seeds**
- **1 tablespoon flaxseeds**
- **Optional toppings: Sliced almonds, fresh berries, and a sprinkle of shredded coconut**

Nutritional Information:

Approximately 220 calories,	*6g protein,*
30g carbohydrates,	*10g fat,*
0mg cholesterol,	*9g fiber,*
650mg potassium,	*120mg sodium.*

1. In a blender, combine the baby spinach, frozen banana, avocado, unsweetened almond milk, chia seeds, and flaxseeds. Blend until smooth and creamy.
2. Taste and adjust the sweetness or thickness by adding more almond milk or a natural sweetener like stevia, if desired.
3. Divide the smoothie mixture into two bowls.
4. Garnish with optional toppings like sliced almonds, fresh berries, and shredded coconut before serving.

This Vegan Green Smoothie Bowl is a nutrient-packed, heart-healthy breakfast or snack. The blend of baby spinach, frozen banana, and avocado provides essential vitamins, minerals, and healthy fats, supporting cardiovascular health. Unsweetened almond milk keeps the smoothie light and cholesterol-free, while chia and flaxseeds add fiber and omega-3 fatty acids, promoting heart health and reducing inflammation. Topped with optional almonds, berries, and shredded coconut, this creamy and delicious smoothie bowl is a perfect way to nourish your heart and start your day with energy.

Steel-Cut Oats with Apple and Cinnamon

Yield: 4 servings | **Prep time:** 5 minutes | **Cook time:** 25 minutes

- **1 cup steel-cut oats**
- **4 cups water**
- **1 large apple, peeled, cored, and diced**
- **2 teaspoons ground cinnamon**
- **1 tablespoon chia seeds (optional)**
- **1 tablespoon maple syrup or honey (optional)**
- **A pinch of salt**

Nutritional Information:

Approximately 210 calories,	*7g protein,*
40g carbohydrates,	*3g fat,*
0mg cholesterol,	*6g fiber,*
115mg potassium,	
10mg sodium.	

1. In a medium saucepan, bring the 4 cups of water to a boil. Add a pinch of salt to the boiling water.
2. Stir in the steel-cut oats and reduce the heat to low. Simmer for 20-25 minutes, stirring occasionally to prevent sticking.
3. While the oats are cooking, dice the apple and add it to a small saucepan with a splash of water and the ground cinnamon. Cook over low heat until the apple pieces are tender.
4. Once the oats are cooked, stir in the cooked apple and cinnamon mixture. If using, add chia seeds and maple syrup or honey for added sweetness and texture.
   Serve hot, optionally garnished with extra slices of apple or a sprinkle of cinnamon.

This Steel-Cut Oats with Apple and Cinnamon recipe is a heart-healthy breakfast option that combines the wholesome goodness of oats with the sweet and spicy flavors of apple and cinnamon. Steel-cut oats provide a rich source of fiber and protein, which help maintain stable blood sugar levels and support heart health. Apples add natural sweetness, vitamins, and additional fiber, while cinnamon offers anti-inflammatory benefits. Optional chia seeds and maple syrup enhance the texture and flavor, making this warm, comforting dish a nutritious and delicious start to your day.

Zucchini Bread Overnight Oats

Yield: 2 servings | **Prep time:** 15 minutes | **Cook time:** 0 minutes (needs to sit overnight)

- **1 cup old-fashioned oats**
- **1 1/2 cups unsweetened almond milk**
- **1 medium zucchini, grated (about 1 cup)**
- **1/2 teaspoon cinnamon**
- **1/4 teaspoon nutmeg**
- **1 tablespoon chia seeds**
- **1 tablespoon flaxseeds**
- **2 teaspoons maple syrup or honey (optional)**
- **Optional toppings: Sliced almonds, fresh berries**

1. In a medium-sized mixing bowl, combine the old-fashioned oats, grated zucchini, cinnamon, nutmeg, chia seeds, and flaxseeds.
2. Pour the unsweetened almond milk over the mixture and stir well to combine.
3. Optionally, add maple syrup or honey for sweetness and mix again.
4. Divide the mixture into two jars or containers with lids. Seal and refrigerate overnight or for at least 6 hours.
5. In the morning, give the oats a good stir and top with optional sliced almonds and fresh berries before eating.

Nutritional Information:

Approximately 250 calories,	*8g protein,*
40g carbohydrates,	*7g fat,*
0mg cholesterol,	*9g fiber,*
350mg potassium,	*100mg sodium.*

Enjoy a heart-healthy breakfast with these Zucchini Bread Overnight Oats. Packed with old-fashioned oats and grated zucchini, this recipe offers fiber and essential nutrients for maintaining cardiovascular health. Unsweetened almond milk keeps it light and cholesterol-free, while chia seeds and flaxseeds provide omega-3 fatty acids, promoting heart health and reducing inflammation. The addition of cinnamon and nutmeg adds a delightful flavor reminiscent of zucchini bread. This easy, make-ahead meal is perfect for busy mornings, ensuring a nutritious and delicious start to your day.

Quinoa Breakfast Bowl with Fresh Fruits

Yield: 2 servings | **Prep time:** 10 minutes | **Cook time:** 15 minutes

- **1 cup quinoa, rinsed and drained**
- **2 cups water**
- **Pinch of salt**
- **1 cup mixed fresh fruits (e.g., sliced banana, berries, apple chunks)**
- **1/2 teaspoon cinnamon**
- **1 tablespoon chia seeds**
- **1 tablespoon flaxseeds**
- **1 tablespoon honey or maple syrup (optional)**
- **Optional toppings: A dollop of Greek yogurt, a sprinkle of nuts**

1. In a medium saucepan, bring the 2 cups of water to a boil. Add a pinch of salt and the quinoa, then reduce the heat to low, cover, and simmer for about 15 minutes or until the quinoa is tender and the water is absorbed.
2. Remove from heat and fluff the quinoa with a fork. Allow it to cool for a few minutes.
3. Stir in the cinnamon, chia seeds, and flaxseeds.
4. Divide the quinoa into two bowls, and top each bowl with the mixed fresh fruits.
5. Drizzle honey or maple syrup over the top for added sweetness, if desired, and garnish with optional toppings like a dollop of Greek yogurt or a sprinkle of nuts.

Nutritional Information:

Approximately 350 calories,	*12g protein,*
55g carbohydrates,	*9g fat,*
0mg cholesterol,	*8g fiber,*
400mg potassium,	*150mg sodium.*

This Quinoa Breakfast Bowl with Fresh Fruits is a nutritious and heart-healthy way to start your day. Quinoa, a high-protein grain, provides essential amino acids and fiber, supporting cardiovascular health and sustained energy. Mixed fresh fruits add natural sweetness and vitamins, while chia and flaxseeds offer omega-3 fatty acids for heart protection. Cinnamon adds a warm, comforting flavor and antioxidants. Optional toppings like Greek yogurt and nuts enhance the nutritional value and taste. This wholesome breakfast bowl is perfect for a balanced and satisfying morning meal.

Kale and Turkey Sausage Breakfast Burrito

Yield: 4 servings | **Prep time:** 15 minutes | **Cook time:** 20 minutes

- **4 whole-grain or whole-wheat tortillas**
- **1 pound lean turkey sausage**
- **1 tablespoon olive oil**
- **4 cups kale, stems removed and chopped**
- **1 medium onion, diced**
- **1 red bell pepper, diced**
- **4 large eggs, beaten (or 1 cup liquid egg whites for lower cholesterol)**
- **Salt and pepper to taste**
- **Optional: Sliced avocado, salsa, low-fat cheese for topping**

Nutritional Information:

180mg cholesterol (will vary if using egg whites),
Approximately 420 calories,   *28g protein,*
40g carbohydrates,   *16g fat,*
720mg sodium,   *6g fiber,*
450mg potassium.

1. In a non-stick skillet over medium heat, cook the turkey sausage, breaking it apart with a spatula, until browned and cooked through. Remove from the skillet and set aside.
2. In the same skillet, add the olive oil, onion, and red bell pepper. Sauté until softened, about 5 minutes.
3. Add the chopped kale to the skillet and continue sautéing until wilted, about 3-5 minutes.
4. Add the beaten eggs (or liquid egg whites) to the skillet, season with salt and pepper, and scramble until cooked. Mix in the cooked turkey sausage.
5. Warm the whole-grain tortillas briefly in the oven or microwave. Divide the skillet mixture among the tortillas, add optional toppings, and roll into burritos.

Start your day with this Kale and Turkey Sausage Breakfast Burrito, packed with heart-healthy ingredients. Lean turkey sausage provides a protein boost without excess fat, while kale offers a rich source of vitamins, fiber, and antioxidants that support cardiovascular health. Whole-grain tortillas and vegetables like onion and red bell pepper add fiber and essential nutrients. Using liquid egg whites can lower cholesterol levels. Optional toppings like avocado and salsa enhance flavor and nutrition. This delicious and nutritious burrito is perfect for a heart-friendly breakfast.

Low-Fat Greek Yogurt Parfait

Yield: 2 servings | **Prep time:** 10 minutes | **Cook time:** 0 minutes

- **2 cups low-fat Greek yogurt**
- **1 cup mixed berries (strawberries, blueberries, raspberries)**
- **1/2 cup granola, low-sugar**
- **1 tablespoon honey or maple syrup (optional)**
- **1 tablespoon chia seeds**
- **1 teaspoon vanilla extract**

Nutritional Information:

Approximately 300 calories,   *20g protein,*
35g carbohydrates,   *8g fat,*
10mg cholesterol,   *5g fiber,*
100mg sodium,

300mg potassium.

1. In a bowl, mix the low-fat Greek yogurt with vanilla extract until well combined.
2. In serving glasses or bowls, layer 1/4 cup of Greek yogurt at the bottom.
3. Add a layer of mixed berries followed by a sprinkle of granola and chia seeds.
4. Repeat the layers, ending with a layer of Greek yogurt on top.
5. Drizzle a small amount of honey or maple syrup over the top if desired.

This Low-Fat Greek Yogurt Parfait is a delightful and heart-healthy way to enjoy a nutritious breakfast or snack. The low-fat Greek yogurt provides a rich source of protein and probiotics, which support heart health and digestion. Mixed berries are packed with antioxidants and fiber, beneficial for reducing inflammation and improving cardiovascular health. The addition of low-sugar granola and chia seeds adds crunch and omega-3 fatty acids, which are vital for heart health. This parfait is easy to assemble and perfect for a refreshing, heart-friendly treat.

Whole-Grain Pancakes with Sugar-Free Maple Syrup

Yield: 4 servings (8 pancakes) | **Prep time:** 10 minutes | **Cook time:** 20 minutes

- **1 1/2 cups whole-grain flour**
- **1 tablespoon baking powder**
- **1/4 teaspoon salt**
- **2 large eggs, beaten**
- **1 1/4 cups skim or almond milk**
- **1 tablespoon olive oil or melted coconut oil**
- **1 teaspoon vanilla extract**
- **Optional: Fresh berries for topping**
- **Sugar-free maple syrup for serving**

Nutritional Information:

Approximately 300 calories,	*10g protein,*
45g carbohydrates,	*8g fat,*
95mg cholesterol,	*7g fiber,*
300mg potassium,	*350mg sodium.*

1. In a large mixing bowl, whisk together the whole-grain flour, baking powder, and salt.
2. In a separate bowl, combine the beaten eggs, skim or almond milk, olive oil, and vanilla extract.
3. Add the wet ingredients to the dry ingredients and stir just until combined; some lumps are okay.
4. Heat a non-stick skillet over medium heat. Use a ladle to pour batter onto the skillet, forming pancakes. Cook until bubbles form on the surface, then flip and cook until the other side is browned.
5. Serve hot with fresh berries and sugar-free maple syrup.

These Whole-Grain Pancakes with Sugar-Free Maple Syrup make for a heart-healthy and satisfying breakfast. Made with whole-grain flour, they provide essential fiber and nutrients that support cardiovascular health. The use of skim or almond milk keeps them low in saturated fat, while olive oil or melted coconut oil adds healthy fats. Topped with fresh berries, these pancakes offer antioxidants and vitamins. Sugar-free maple syrup ensures a sweet finish without the added sugars, making this dish a perfect.

Smoked Salmon and Cucumber Bagel (Whole Grain)

Yield: 2 servings | **Prep time:** 10 minutes | **Cook time:** 0 minutes

- **2 whole-grain bagels, halved**
- **4 ounces smoked salmon**
- **1 medium cucumber, thinly sliced**
- **1/2 cup low-fat cream cheese**
- **1 tablespoon capers (optional)**
- **Fresh dill for garnish (optional)**
- **Salt and pepper to taste**

Nutritional Information:

Approximately 360 calories,	*20g protein,*
45g carbohydrates,	*10g fat,*
20mg cholesterol,	*6g fiber,*
540mg sodium,	

320mg potassium.

1. Toast the whole-grain bagels until they are lightly crispy.
2. Spread a layer of low-fat cream cheese on the cut side of each bagel half.
3. Arrange cucumber slices over the cream cheese, followed by smoked salmon.
4. If using, sprinkle capers over the smoked salmon and add a garnish of fresh dill.
5. Season with a pinch of salt and pepper to taste, then serve immediately.

This Smoked Salmon and Cucumber Bagel is a heart-healthy, protein-rich breakfast or lunch option. Whole-grain bagels provide essential fiber and nutrients, supporting heart health and digestion. Smoked salmon is rich in omega-3 fatty acids, which are beneficial for cardiovascular health. The combination of low-fat cream cheese and fresh cucumber adds a light, creamy texture and refreshing crunch. Optional capers and dill enhance the flavor without adding unnecessary calories. Enjoy this nutritious and delicious bagel for a balanced meal that promotes heart health.

Raspberry and Chia Seed Smoothie

Yield: 2 servings | Prep time: 5 minutes | Cook time: 0 minutes

- **1 cup frozen raspberries**
- **1 banana, peeled and sliced**
- **1 tablespoon chia seeds**
- **1 cup almond milk (unsweetened)**
- **1/2 cup Greek yogurt (non-fat)**
- **1 teaspoon honey or a sugar substitute (optional)**

Nutritional Information:

Approximately 160 calories,	8g protein,
28g carbohydrates,	3g fat,
0mg cholesterol,	9g fiber,
320mg potassium,	90mg sodium.

1. Place the frozen raspberries, banana slices, chia seeds, almond milk, and Greek yogurt into a blender.
2. Blend on high speed until smooth. If the mixture is too thick, add a bit more almond milk to reach your desired consistency.
3. Taste the smoothie and add honey or a sugar substitute if you prefer it sweeter. Blend again briefly to mix.
4. Pour the smoothie into two glasses and serve immediately.

This Raspberry and Chia Seed Smoothie is a refreshing and heart-healthy choice, perfect for a quick breakfast or snack. Packed with antioxidants from raspberries and fiber from chia seeds, this smoothie supports cardiovascular health and digestion. The banana adds natural sweetness and potassium, essential for maintaining healthy blood pressure. Non-fat Greek yogurt provides a protein boost without added fat, while unsweetened almond milk keeps it light and creamy. Enjoy this delicious and nutritious smoothie for a heart-friendly treat any time of day.

Blueberry and Flaxseed Muffins

Yield: 12 muffins | Prep time: 15 minutes | Cook time: 25 minutes

- **1 1/2 cups whole-grain flour**
- **1/2 cup ground flaxseed**
- **1/2 cup old-fashioned oats**
- **2 teaspoons baking powder**
- **1/2 teaspoon baking soda**
- **1/4 teaspoon salt**
- **1/2 cup unsweetened applesauce**
- **1/4 cup olive oil or melted coconut oil**
- **1/2 cup almond milk or other plant-based milk**
- **1/4 cup maple syrup or honey**
- **1 teaspoon vanilla extract**
- **1 cup fresh blueberries**

Nutritional Information:

Approximately 160 calories,	4g protein,
25g carbohydrates,	5g fat,
0mg cholesterol,	4g fiber,
220mg sodium,	90mg potassium.

1. Preheat your oven to 350°F (175°C). Line a muffin pan with paper liners or grease the pan with a little oil.
2. In a large mixing bowl, combine whole-grain flour, ground flaxseed, oats, baking powder, baking soda, and salt.
3. In a separate bowl, whisk together unsweetened applesauce, olive oil, almond milk, maple syrup, and vanilla extract.
4. Fold the wet ingredients into the dry ingredients until just combined. Do not overmix. Gently fold in the blueberries.
5. Divide the batter evenly among the prepared muffin cups. Bake for 25 minutes or until a toothpick inserted into the center comes out clean.

These Blueberry and Flaxseed Muffins are a heart-healthy treat perfect for breakfast or a snack. Made with whole-grain flour and ground flaxseed, they offer a boost of fiber and omega-3 fatty acids, supporting cardiovascular health. Fresh blueberries add antioxidants and natural sweetness, while unsweetened applesauce and almond milk keep the muffins moist and low in saturated fat. Sweetened with maple syrup or honey, these muffins are delicious and nutritious, making them an ideal addition to a heart-friendly diet. Enjoy their wholesome goodness any time of the day.

Chickpea Scramble Tofu Wrap

Yield: 4 servings | **Prep time:** 15 minutes | **Cook time:** 20 minutes

- 1 cup chickpeas, drained and rinsed
- 1 block (14 oz) firm tofu, drained and crumbled
- 1 tablespoon olive oil
- 1 medium onion, diced
- 1 bell pepper, diced
- 1 teaspoon turmeric powder
- 1 teaspoon garlic powder
- Salt and pepper to taste
- 4 whole-grain tortillas
- 1 cup fresh spinach leaves
- Optional: salsa or hot sauce for serving

Nutritional Information:

Approximately 420 calories,	18g protein,
60g carbohydrates,	12g fat,
0mg cholesterol,	10g fiber
450mg potassium,	700mg sodium.

1. In a skillet, heat the olive oil over medium heat. Add the diced onion and bell pepper, cooking until softened.
2. Add crumbled tofu, chickpeas, turmeric, and garlic powder to the skillet. Stir well, breaking apart the tofu as you go, and cook until heated through. Season with salt and pepper to taste.
3. Warm the whole-grain tortillas in a separate pan or directly over a gas flame for about 10-15 seconds on each side.
4. Assemble the wraps: Place a generous amount of the chickpea-tofu scramble in the center of each tortilla. Top with fresh spinach leaves.
5. Fold the sides of the tortilla over the filling, then roll up from the bottom to make a wrap. Cut in half and serve immediately, optionally with salsa or hot sauce.

This Chickpea Scramble Tofu Wrap is a delicious and heart-healthy meal perfect for any time of day. The combination of chickpeas and tofu provides a rich source of plant-based protein and fiber, which are essential for cardiovascular health. Turmeric adds anti-inflammatory benefits, while fresh spinach offers vital vitamins and minerals. Wrapped in whole-grain tortillas, this dish supports digestive health and sustains energy levels. Enjoy these flavorful wraps with optional salsa or hot sauce for an extra kick, making them a nutritious and satisfying choice.

Coconut and Matcha Chia Pudding

Yield: 4 servings | **Prep time:** 10 minutes | **Cook time:** 0 minutes (Refrigeration time: 4 hours)

- 1/4 cup chia seeds
- 1 can (13.5 oz) light coconut milk
- 1 tablespoon matcha powder
- 1 tablespoon maple syrup or agave nectar
- 1 teaspoon vanilla extract
- Fresh fruits for garnish (optional)

Nutritional Information:

Approximately 200 calories,	4g protein,
15g carbohydrates,	14g fat,
0mg cholesterol,	10g fiber,
80mg sodium,	
240mg potassium.	

1. In a medium-sized mixing bowl, whisk together the light coconut milk, matcha powder, maple syrup, and vanilla extract until well combined.
2. Add chia seeds to the liquid mixture and stir thoroughly to prevent clumping.
3. Cover the bowl and place it in the refrigerator for at least 4 hours, or overnight for best results.
4. Before serving, give the pudding a good stir to distribute any settled chia seeds evenly.
5. Divide the pudding into 4 servings, garnish with fresh fruits if desired, and enjoy!

This Coconut and Matcha Chia Pudding is a delightful and heart-healthy dessert or snack. Chia seeds provide a rich source of omega-3 fatty acids, fiber, and protein, which support cardiovascular health and digestion. Light coconut milk adds a creamy texture without excess calories, while matcha powder offers antioxidants and a subtle, energizing flavor. Sweetened with a touch of maple syrup and vanilla extract, this pudding is both nutritious and delicious. Garnish with fresh fruits for added vitamins and enjoy this refreshing, heart-friendly treat.

Sweet Potato Hash with Black Beans

Yield: 4 servings | **Prep time:** 15 minutes | **Cook time:** 25 minutes

- 2 medium sweet potatoes, peeled and diced
- 1 can (15 ounces) black beans, drained and rinsed
- 1 medium onion, finely chopped
- 2 cloves garlic, minced
- 1 medium red bell pepper, diced
- 2 tablespoons olive oil
- 1 teaspoon ground cumin
- 1/2 teaspoon paprika
- 1/4 teaspoon cayenne pepper (optional, for heat)
- Salt and pepper to taste
- Fresh cilantro for garnish (optional)

Nutritional Information:

Approximately 275 calories,	*8g protein,*
45g carbohydrates,	*7g fat,*
0mg cholesterol,	*10g fiber,*
800mg potassium,	*300mg sodium.*

1. Preheat the oven to 400°F (200°C). Place diced sweet potatoes on a baking sheet, drizzle with 1 tablespoon olive oil, sprinkle with cumin, paprika, salt, and pepper. Toss to coat and bake for 20-25 minutes, or until tender.
2. While the sweet potatoes are baking, heat the remaining 1 tablespoon olive oil in a large skillet over medium heat. Add the onions and garlic, and sauté until translucent, about 5 minutes.
3. Stir in the diced red bell pepper and cook for another 2-3 minutes. Add the drained and rinsed black beans, and heat through.
Once the sweet potatoes are done, add them to the skillet and mix everything well. Adjust the seasoning if necessary and garnish with fresh cilantro before serving.

This Sweet Potato Hash with Black Beans is a delicious and heart-healthy dish, perfect for any meal. Sweet potatoes are rich in fiber, vitamins, and potassium, which help regulate blood pressure and support heart health. Black beans provide plant-based protein and additional fiber, aiding in cholesterol management. The blend of cumin, paprika, and optional cayenne pepper adds a flavorful kick, while olive oil ensures healthy fats. Garnished with fresh cilantro, this vibrant and nutritious hash is a wholesome addition to a heart-friendly diet. Enjoy its delightful taste and benefits for your heart.

Nut Butter and Banana Breakfast Sandwich

Yield: 2 servings | **Prep time:** 10 minutes | **Cook time:** 5 minutes

- 4 slices of whole-grain bread
- 2 tablespoons almond butter or any other heart-healthy nut butter
- 2 medium bananas, sliced
- 1 tablespoon chia seeds
- 1 teaspoon honey or maple syrup (optional)
- A pinch of cinnamon (optional)

Nutritional Information:

Approximately 300 calories,	*9g protein,*
50g carbohydrates,	*10g fat,*
0mg cholesterol,	*9g fiber,*
600mg potassium,	*200mg sodium.*

1. Toast the whole-grain bread slices until they reach your desired level of crispiness.
2. Spread 1 tablespoon of almond butter evenly on one side of two slices of the toasted bread.
3. Place sliced bananas over the almond butter, and sprinkle chia seeds on top.
4. If using, drizzle a small amount of honey or maple syrup and add a pinch of cinnamon over the bananas.
5. Close the sandwiches with the remaining slices of bread, press lightly, and serve immediately.

This Nut Butter and Banana Breakfast Sandwich is a heart-healthy, quick, and delicious way to start your day. Whole-grain bread provides essential fiber and nutrients, while almond butter offers healthy fats and protein, beneficial for cardiovascular health. Bananas add natural sweetness and potassium, crucial for maintaining healthy blood pressure. Chia seeds contribute additional fiber and omega-3 fatty acids, enhancing heart protection. A drizzle of honey or maple syrup and a pinch of cinnamon can be added for extra flavor. Enjoy this nutritious and satisfying sandwich for a wholesome breakfast.

Veggie-Loaded Breakfast Casserole

Yield: 6 servings | **Prep time:** 15 minutes | **Cook time:** 45 minutes

- **8 large eggs**
- **1 cup skim milk**
- **1 medium onion, diced**
- **1 bell pepper, diced**
- **1 medium zucchini, diced**
- **1 cup spinach, chopped**
- **1 cup cherry tomatoes, halved**
- **1/2 cup low-fat shredded cheese (e.g., cheddar or mozzarella)**
- **1 teaspoon olive oil**
- **Salt and pepper to taste**

Nutritional Information:

Approximately 160 calories,	*12g protein,*
8g carbohydrates,	*8g fat,*
210mg cholesterol,	*2g fiber,*
360mg potassium,	*220mg sodium.*

1. Preheat your oven to 375°F (190°C). Grease a 9x13-inch casserole dish with olive oil.
2. In a large bowl, whisk together the eggs, skim milk, salt, and pepper.
3. In a skillet over medium heat, sauté the diced onion, bell pepper, and zucchini until soft. Add the chopped spinach just to wilt, then remove from heat.
4. Arrange the sautéed veggies and halved cherry tomatoes in the greased casserole dish. Pour the egg mixture over the veggies.
5. Sprinkle the shredded cheese on top and bake for 45 minutes, or until the eggs are set and the top is lightly golden.

This Veggie-Loaded Breakfast Casserole is a heart-healthy, nutrient-packed way to start your day. With a mix of fresh vegetables like zucchini, spinach, and bell peppers, it provides essential vitamins, minerals, and fiber that support cardiovascular health. The eggs and low-fat cheese offer high-quality protein without excessive fat, while skim milk keeps it light and creamy. This casserole is both satisfying and nutritious, making it an excellent choice for a balanced breakfast that promotes heart health. Enjoy it warm for a delightful and healthy morning meal.

Buckwheat and Berry Smoothie

Yield: 2 servings | **Prep time:** 10 minutes | **Cook time:** 0 minutes

- **1/2 cup buckwheat groats, soaked overnight and drained**
- **1 cup mixed berries (strawberries, blueberries, raspberries)**
- **1 medium banana**
- **1 tablespoon chia seeds**
- **1 tablespoon flaxseeds**
- **1 cup unsweetened almond milk**
- **1 teaspoon honey or maple syrup (optional)**
- **Ice cubes (optional)**

Nutritional Information:

Approximately 220 calories,	*8g protein,*
40g carbohydrates,	*6g fat,*
0mg cholesterol,	*10g fiber,*
450mg potassium,	*90mg sodium.*

1. Place soaked and drained buckwheat groats, mixed berries, banana, chia seeds, and flaxseeds in a blender.
2. Add unsweetened almond milk to the blender.
3. If using, add honey or maple syrup for extra sweetness.
4. Blend on high speed until smooth, adding ice cubes if a colder smoothie is desired.
5. Pour into glasses and serve immediately.

This Buckwheat and Berry Smoothie is a heart-healthy, nutrient-rich option perfect for breakfast or a snack. Soaked buckwheat groats add a unique texture and are packed with fiber and protein, supporting cardiovascular health and digestion. Mixed berries provide antioxidants and natural sweetness, while banana contributes potassium essential for blood pressure regulation. Chia and flaxseeds boost omega-3 fatty acids, enhancing heart protection. Unsweetened almond milk keeps it light and creamy. Enjoy this delicious smoothie for a refreshing and wholesome start to your day.

Shakshuka with Spinach and Chickpeas

Yield: 4 servings | **Prep time:** 10 minutes | **Cook time:** 20 minutes

- **2 tablespoons olive oil**
- **1 medium onion, chopped**
- **3 cloves garlic, minced**
- **1 can (15 oz) chickpeas, drained and rinsed**
- **1 can (14 oz) diced tomatoes**
- **2 cups fresh spinach leaves**
- **4 large eggs**
- **1 teaspoon paprika**
- **1 teaspoon cumin**
- **Salt and pepper to taste**
- **Fresh parsley, for garnish (optional)**

Nutritional Information:

Approximately 320 calories,	*16g protein,*
40g carbohydrates,	*12g fat,*
186mg cholesterol,	*9g fiber,*
800mg potassium,	*600mg sodium.*

1. In a large skillet, heat olive oil over medium heat. Add chopped onion and garlic, and sauté until translucent.
2. Add chickpeas, diced tomatoes (with juice), paprika, and cumin. Stir well to combine and let simmer for about 5-7 minutes.
3. Stir in the spinach leaves until wilted, making sure the mixture is evenly spread across the skillet.
4. Create four small wells in the mixture and crack an egg into each well. Cover the skillet and cook until the eggs are done to your liking (about 5-7 minutes for runny yolks).
5. Season with salt and pepper to taste. Garnish with fresh parsley, if desired, before serving.

This Shakshuka with Spinach and Chickpeas is a flavorful and heart-healthy dish perfect for breakfast or brunch. The combination of chickpeas and spinach provides a high-fiber, nutrient-dense base rich in vitamins, minerals, and plant-based protein, supporting cardiovascular health. The eggs add additional protein and essential nutrients. Seasoned with paprika and cumin, this dish offers a warm and savory flavor profile. Topped with fresh parsley, this vibrant and wholesome meal is both satisfying and nutritious, making it an excellent choice for a heart-friendly diet.

Baked Avocado Eggs with Fresh Salsa

Yield: 4 servings | **Prep time:** 10 minutes | **Cook time:** 15 minutes

- **2 large avocados, halved and pitted**
- **4 small eggs**
- **Salt and pepper to taste**
- **1 cup fresh salsa (homemade or store-bought)**
- **1 tablespoon chopped cilantro (optional)**
- **1 lime, cut into wedges (optional)**

Nutritional Information:

Approximately 230 calories,	*8g protein,*
12g carbohydrates,	*18g fat,*
186mg cholesterol,	*7g fiber,*
700mg potassium,	*420mg sodium.*

1. Preheat the oven to 425°F (220°C). Scoop out some flesh from the avocado halves to make enough room for the eggs.
2. Place the avocado halves in a baking dish. Carefully crack an egg into each avocado half. Season with salt and pepper.
3. Bake for 12-15 minutes or until the eggs are cooked to your liking.
4. Spoon fresh salsa over the baked avocado eggs and garnish with chopped cilantro and a lime wedge, if desired.

These Baked Avocado Eggs with Fresh Salsa are a delicious and heart-healthy breakfast or brunch option. Avocados provide healthy monounsaturated fats, fiber, and potassium, which are essential for cardiovascular health. The eggs add high-quality protein and essential nutrients. Topped with fresh salsa, this dish brings a burst of flavor and antioxidants, enhancing its nutritional value. Garnish with cilantro and lime wedges for an extra fresh taste. This satisfying and nutritious meal supports heart health while delighting your taste buds. Enjoy this wholesome and flavorful dish for a perfect start to your day.

Tofu Benedict with Avocado Sauce

Yield: 4 servings | **Prep time:** 15 minutes | **Cook time:** 10 minutes

- **1 block (14 oz) firm tofu, drained and pressed**
- **2 tablespoons olive oil**
- **4 whole-grain English muffins, split and toasted**
- **2 cups baby spinach**
- **1 ripe avocado**
- **1/4 cup unsweetened almond milk**
- **1 tablespoon lemon juice**
- **Salt and pepper to taste**
- **Paprika for garnish (optional)**

Nutritional Information:

Approximately 380 calories,	*21g protein,*
35g carbohydrates,	*18g fat,*
0mg cholesterol,	*9g fiber,*
600mg potassium,	*400mg sodium.*

1. Cut the tofu block into 8 even slices. Heat the olive oil in a skillet over medium heat and cook the tofu slices for 3-4 minutes per side until golden brown. Set aside.
2. In a blender, combine the avocado, almond milk, and lemon juice. Blend until smooth. Season the avocado sauce with salt and pepper to taste.
3. To assemble the benedict, place a handful of baby spinach on each toasted English muffin half. Top with a slice of tofu.
4. Drizzle the avocado sauce over the tofu and garnish with a sprinkle of paprika, if desired.

This Tofu Benedict with Avocado Sauce is a heart-healthy and delicious twist on a classic breakfast dish. Firm tofu provides a high-protein, low-fat alternative to traditional eggs, while whole-grain English muffins add fiber and essential nutrients. Baby spinach offers a boost of vitamins and minerals, and the creamy avocado sauce, made with almond milk and lemon juice, provides healthy monounsaturated fats and antioxidants. Garnished with paprika, this flavorful and nutritious meal supports cardiovascular health, making it a perfect choice for a wholesome breakfast or brunch.

HEART HEALTHY

— ★★★★★ —

DIET

Chapter

6

Salads

Chickpea and Roasted Veggie Medley

Yield: 4 servings | **Prep time:** 15 minutes | **Cook time:** 25 minutes

- **1 can (15 ounces) chickpeas, drained and rinsed**
- **2 cups broccoli florets**
- **1 red bell pepper, cut into strips**
- **1 zucchini, sliced into half-moons**
- **1 medium red onion, sliced**
- **2 tablespoons olive oil**
- **1 teaspoon paprika**
- **1/2 teaspoon garlic powder**
- **Salt and pepper to taste**
- **Optional: A pinch of red pepper flakes for heat**
- **Optional: Fresh parsley for garnish**

1. Preheat your oven to 400°F (200°C). Line a baking sheet with parchment paper.
2. In a large bowl, combine chickpeas, broccoli, red bell pepper, zucchini, and red onion.
3. Drizzle olive oil over the vegetables and chickpeas. Add paprika, garlic powder, salt, and pepper. Toss everything to coat evenly.
4. Spread the mixture onto the prepared baking sheet in a single layer. Roast in the oven for 25 minutes, or until the veggies are tender and slightly browned.
5. Optional: Garnish with fresh parsley and red pepper flakes before serving.

Nutritional Information:

Approximately 250 calories,	10g protein,
35g carbohydrates,	8g fat,
0mg cholesterol,	9g fiber,
600mg potassium,	300mg sodium.

This Chickpea and Roasted Veggie Medley is a heart-healthy, nutrient-packed dish perfect for any meal. Chickpeas provide plant-based protein and fiber, supporting cardiovascular health and digestion. The mix of broccoli, red bell pepper, zucchini, and red onion offers a variety of vitamins, minerals, and antioxidants. Olive oil adds healthy fats, while paprika and garlic powder enhance the flavor. Optional red pepper flakes add a spicy kick, and fresh parsley provides a fresh garnish. This colorful and delicious medley is both satisfying and nutritious, making it an excellent choice for a balanced diet.

Grilled Salmon and Asparagus Salad

Yield: 4 servings | **Prep time:** 20 minutes | **Cook time:** 15 minutes

- 4 salmon fillets (4-6 ounces each)
- 1 bunch asparagus, trimmed
- 1 tablespoon olive oil
- Salt and pepper to taste
- 6 cups mixed greens (e.g., spinach, arugula, romaine)
- 1 cup cherry tomatoes, halved
- 1 avocado, sliced
- 1/4 cup red onion, thinly sliced

For the Dressing:
- 2 tablespoons extra virgin olive oil
- 1 tablespoon lemon juice
- Salt and pepper to taste

Nutritional Information:

Approximately 450 calories,	35g protein,
20g carbohydrates,	25g fat,
70mg cholesterol,	8g fiber,
950mg potassium,	150mg sodium.

1. Preheat your grill to medium-high heat.
2. Rub the salmon fillets and asparagus with 1 tablespoon of olive oil, and season with salt and pepper.
3. Grill the salmon and asparagus for about 5-7 minutes per side, or until the salmon is cooked to your desired level and the asparagus is tender yet crisp.
4. While the salmon and asparagus are grilling, prepare the salad by combining the mixed greens, cherry tomatoes, avocado, and red onion in a large bowl.
5. Whisk together the dressing ingredients and toss the salad with the dressing. Once the salmon and asparagus are done, place them on top of the salad and serve immediately.

This Grilled Salmon and Asparagus Salad is a heart-healthy and nutrient-rich meal. Salmon is packed with omega-3 fatty acids, which support cardiovascular health, while asparagus provides fiber, vitamins, and antioxidants. Mixed greens, cherry tomatoes, and avocado add a variety of essential nutrients and healthy fats. The simple lemon-olive oil dressing enhances the flavors without adding unnecessary calories. This salad is both delicious and satisfying, making it an excellent choice for a balanced diet and a great way to enjoy a nutritious meal.

Spinach and Strawberry Summer Salad

Yield: 4 servings | **Prep time:** 15 minutes | **Cook time:** 0 minutes

- 6 cups fresh baby spinach
- 2 cups strawberries, hulled and sliced
- 1/4 cup almonds, sliced
- 1/2 red onion, thinly sliced
- 1/4 cup feta cheese, crumbled (optional)
- 2 tablespoons extra-virgin olive oil
- 1 tablespoon balsamic vinegar
- Salt and pepper to taste

Nutritional Information:

Approximately 200 calories,	6g protein,
12g carbohydrates,	15g fat,
5mg cholesterol (if feta is used),	4g fiber,
450mg potassium,	150mg sodium.

1. In a large bowl, combine the baby spinach, sliced strawberries, and thinly sliced red onion.
2. In a separate small bowl, whisk together the extra-virgin olive oil and balsamic vinegar. Season with salt and pepper to taste.
3. Pour the dressing over the salad mixture and gently toss to coat all the ingredients evenly.
4. Top the salad with sliced almonds and optional feta cheese before serving.

This Spinach and Strawberry Summer Salad is a refreshing and heart-healthy dish, perfect for warm weather. Fresh baby spinach provides a rich source of vitamins and antioxidants, supporting cardiovascular health. Strawberries add natural sweetness and additional antioxidants, while sliced almonds contribute healthy fats and protein. The thinly sliced red onion offers a subtle bite, and optional feta cheese adds a creamy texture. Tossed with a simple dressing of extra-virgin olive oil and balsamic vinegar, this salad is both delicious and nutritious, making it an ideal choice for a light and healthy meal.

Curried Lentil and Mixed Greens Salad

Yield: 4 servings | **Prep time:** 20 minutes | **Cook time:** 30 minutes

- 1 cup dry green lentils, rinsed and drained
- 4 cups mixed salad greens (spinach, arugula, romaine, etc.)
- 1 medium carrot, shredded
- 1 small red onion, thinly sliced
- 1 bell pepper, diced
- 1 tablespoon olive oil
- 1 teaspoon curry powder
- Salt and pepper to taste (use salt sparingly for a heart-healthy option)

Dressing:
- 2 tablespoons olive oil
- 1 tablespoon lemon juice
- 1 teaspoon Dijon mustard
- 1 teaspoon honey or maple syrup (for a vegan option)

Nutritional Information:

Approximately 280 calories,	*13g protein,*
40g carbohydrates,	*8g fat,*
0mg cholesterol,	*12g fiber*
600mg potassium,	*80mg sodium.*

1. In a medium saucepan, combine lentils with 3 cups of water. Bring to a boil, then reduce heat to low and simmer for 25-30 minutes, or until lentils are tender but not mushy. Drain and let cool.
2. In a large mixing bowl, combine cooked lentils, mixed greens, shredded carrot, diced bell pepper, and thinly sliced red onion.
3. In a small pan, heat 1 tablespoon of olive oil over medium heat. Add curry powder and sauté for 1-2 minutes until fragrant. Add the curried oil to the salad mixture and toss well.
4. In a small bowl, whisk together the dressing ingredients: olive oil, lemon juice, Dijon mustard, and honey or maple syrup. Pour the dressing over the salad and toss to combine.

This Curried Lentil and Mixed Greens Salad is a flavorful and heart-healthy dish. Green lentils provide a rich source of protein and fiber, supporting cardiovascular health and digestion. Mixed salad greens, such as spinach, arugula, and romaine, offer a variety of vitamins and antioxidants. Shredded carrot, red onion, and bell pepper add crunch and additional nutrients. The curry powder adds a warm, aromatic flavor, while the lemon-Dijon dressing ties everything together with a tangy touch. This nutritious and satisfying salad is perfect for a balanced diet, promoting overall heart health.

Cucumber, Mint, and Watermelon Hydration Salad

Yield: 4 servings | **Prep time:** 10 minutes | **Cook time:** 0 minutes

- 4 cups watermelon, cubed
- 2 cups cucumber, sliced
- 1/4 cup fresh mint leaves, chopped
- Juice of 1 lime
- A pinch of salt
- Optional: 1 tablespoon honey or agave syrup for sweetness

Nutritional Information:

Approximately 60 calories,	*1g protein,*
15g carbohydrates,	*0g fat,*
0mg cholesterol,	*1g fiber,*
200mg potassium,	*30mg sodium.*

1. In a large bowl, combine the watermelon and cucumber slices.
2. In a separate bowl, mix the lime juice, chopped mint, and a pinch of salt. Add honey or agave syrup if using.
3. Pour the lime-mint dressing over the watermelon and cucumber mixture.
4. Toss the salad gently to mix the ingredients well and coat them with the dressing.
5. Serve immediately or chill in the refrigerator for 15-20 minutes before serving for best flavor.

This Cucumber, Mint, and Watermelon Hydration Salad is a refreshing and heart-healthy dish perfect for hot days. Watermelon and cucumber provide hydration and essential vitamins, while fresh mint adds a burst of flavor and cooling effect. The lime juice dressing enhances the taste with a tangy note, and a pinch of salt brings out the natural sweetness of the fruits. Optional honey or agave syrup can add extra sweetness. This low-calorie, nutrient-rich salad is perfect for maintaining hydration and supporting heart health. Enjoy chilled for the best flavor.

Mediterranean Farro Salad with Lemon-Tahini Dressing

Yield: 4 servings | **Prep time:** 20 minutes | **Cook time:** 30 minutes

- **1 cup farro, uncooked**
- **4 cups water (for boiling farro)**
- **1 cup cherry tomatoes, halved**
- **1 cucumber, diced**
- **1 red bell pepper, diced**
- **1/2 cup Kalamata olives, pitted and sliced**
- **1/4 cup red onion, finely chopped**
- **1/4 cup fresh parsley, chopped**

For the Lemon-Tahini Dressing:
- **1/4 cup tahini**
- **2 tablespoons lemon juice**
- **1 garlic clove, minced**
- **Salt and pepper to taste**
- **2-4 tablespoons water (to thin the dressing)**

Nutritional Information:
Approximately 350 calories,   *9g protein,*
55g carbohydrates,   *12g fat,*
0mg cholesterol,   *10g fiber,*
450mg potassium,   *250mg sodium.*

1. In a large pot, bring 4 cups of water to a boil. Add the farro and cook according to package directions, usually about 25-30 minutes, until tender but still chewy. Drain and set aside to cool.
2. In a large bowl, combine the cooked farro, cherry tomatoes, cucumber, red bell pepper, Kalamata olives, red onion, and parsley.
3. In a small bowl, whisk together the tahini, lemon juice, minced garlic, salt, and pepper. Add water to reach your desired consistency.
4. Pour the Lemon-Tahini Dressing over the farro and veggie mixture and toss well to combine.
5. Serve immediately or let it chill in the fridge for about 30 minutes to allow the flavors to meld together.

This Mediterranean Farro Salad with Lemon-Tahini Dressing is a flavorful and heart-healthy dish. Farro is an ancient grain rich in fiber and protein, supporting cardiovascular health and digestion. The salad includes cherry tomatoes, cucumber, red bell pepper, Kalamata olives, red onion, and parsley, offering a variety of vitamins, minerals, and antioxidants. The creamy lemon-tahini dressing adds a tangy and rich flavor while providing healthy fats. This refreshing and nutritious salad is perfect for a light lunch or dinner, promoting overall well-being and heart health.

Avocado and Pomegranate Seed Salad

Yield: 4 servings | **Prep time:** 15 minutes | **Cook time:** 0 minutes

- **2 ripe avocados, peeled, pitted, and cubed**
- **1 cup pomegranate seeds**
- **4 cups mixed salad greens (e.g., spinach, arugula, romaine)**
- **1/4 cup walnuts, toasted**
- **Juice of 1 lemon**
- **2 tablespoons olive oil**
- **Salt and pepper to taste**

Nutritional Information:
Approximately 280 calories,   *4g protein,*
18g carbohydrates,   *24g fat,*
0mg cholesterol,   *8g fiber,*
400mg potassium,   *10mg sodium.*

1. In a large salad bowl, combine the mixed greens, avocado cubes, and pomegranate seeds.
2. In a small bowl, whisk together the lemon juice, olive oil, salt, and pepper to create the dressing.
3. Drizzle the dressing over the salad and toss gently to combine all the ingredients.
4. Top the salad with toasted walnuts before serving.

This Avocado and Pomegranate Seed Salad is a vibrant and heart-healthy dish perfect for any meal. Avocados provide healthy monounsaturated fats, fiber, and potassium, which are essential for cardiovascular health. Pomegranate seeds add a burst of sweetness and are rich in antioxidants. Mixed greens offer a variety of vitamins and minerals, while toasted walnuts contribute omega-3 fatty acids. The lemon-olive oil dressing enhances the flavors with a tangy and refreshing touch. Enjoy this delicious and nutritious salad for a heart-friendly and satisfying meal.

Kale and Quinoa Superfood Salad

Yield: 4 servings | **Prep time:** 20 minutes | **Cook time:** 15 minutes

- 1 cup quinoa, rinsed
- 2 cups water
- 4 cups kale, destemmed and chopped
- 1 cup cherry tomatoes, halved
- 1 avocado, diced
- 1/2 cup walnuts, chopped
- 1/4 cup dried cranberries
- 1 tablespoon olive oil
- Juice of 1 lemon
- Salt and pepper to taste

Nutritional Information:

Approximately 400 calories,
45g carbohydrates,
0mg cholesterol,
700mg potassium,
12g protein,
20g fat,
8g fiber,
50mg sodium.

1. In a medium saucepan, bring 2 cups of water to a boil. Add the quinoa, reduce heat to low, cover, and cook for 15 minutes or until quinoa is cooked and water is absorbed. Fluff with a fork and let it cool.
2. In a large bowl, massage the chopped kale with olive oil until the leaves become tender.
3. Add the cooked and cooled quinoa to the kale along with the cherry tomatoes, diced avocado, chopped walnuts, and dried cranberries.
4. Squeeze lemon juice over the salad and toss to combine. Season with salt and pepper to taste.

This Kale and Quinoa Superfood Salad is a nutrient-dense, heart-healthy meal perfect for any time of day. Quinoa provides a complete protein and is rich in fiber, supporting cardiovascular health. Kale, a superfood, is packed with vitamins, minerals, and antioxidants. Cherry tomatoes add a burst of flavor and additional vitamins, while avocado offers healthy fats. Walnuts contribute omega-3 fatty acids, and dried cranberries provide a touch of natural sweetness. Tossed with olive oil and lemon juice, this salad is both delicious and nutritious, promoting overall heart health.

Southwest Black Bean and Corn Salad

Yield: 4 servings | **Prep time:** 15 minutes | **Cook time:** 0 minutes

- 1 can (15 oz) black beans, drained and rinsed
- 1 can (15 oz) corn kernels, drained and rinsed
- 1 red bell pepper, diced
- 1 avocado, diced
- 1/4 cup red onion, finely chopped
- 1/4 cup fresh cilantro, chopped
- 1 lime, juiced
- 1 tablespoon olive oil
- Salt and pepper to taste

Nutritional Information:

Approximately 250 calories,
35g carbohydrates,
0mg cholesterol,
8g protein,
10g fat,
11g fiber,
600mg potassium,
400mg sodium.

1. In a large bowl, combine the black beans, corn kernels, red bell pepper, avocado, and red onion.
2. In a small bowl, whisk together the lime juice, olive oil, salt, and pepper.
3. Pour the dressing over the salad ingredients and mix well to combine.
4. Fold in the chopped cilantro.
5. Serve immediately or refrigerate for about 30 minutes to allow the flavors to meld together.

This Southwest Black Bean and Corn Salad is a vibrant, heart-healthy dish packed with flavor and nutrition. Black beans provide a rich source of plant-based protein and fiber, supporting cardiovascular health and digestion. Corn adds sweetness and additional fiber, while red bell pepper and red onion offer vitamins and antioxidants. Avocado contributes healthy fats, and fresh cilantro enhances the flavor. The lime juice and olive oil dressing add a zesty, refreshing touch. Enjoy this salad as a light meal or a side dish, perfect for a heart-friendly diet.

Spicy Thai Mango and Tofu Salad

Yield: 4 servings | **Prep time:** 20 minutes | **Cook time:** 10 minutes

- **1 block (14 oz.) firm tofu, drained and cut into 1-inch cubes**
- **1 large mango, peeled and diced**
- **4 cups mixed salad greens (e.g., spinach, arugula, romaine)**
- **1 medium red bell pepper, thinly sliced**
- **1 small red onion, thinly sliced**
- **1/4 cup fresh cilantro leaves, chopped**
- **2 tablespoons fresh mint leaves, chopped**

For the dressing:
- **2 tablespoons low-sodium soy sauce**
- **1 tablespoon rice vinegar**
- **1 tablespoon freshly squeezed lime juice**
- **1 teaspoon sesame oil**
- **1 teaspoon chili flakes (adjust to taste)**

1. In a non-stick skillet over medium heat, cook the tofu cubes until they turn golden brown on all sides. Remove from heat and set aside.
2. In a large bowl, combine the cooked tofu, diced mango, mixed salad greens, red bell pepper, red onion, cilantro, and mint leaves.
3. In a small bowl, whisk together all the dressing ingredients until well combined.
4. Drizzle the dressing over the salad and gently toss to combine. Serve immediately.

Nutritional Information:

Approximately 250 calories,	*14g protein,*
32g carbohydrates,	*8g fat,*
0mg cholesterol,	*6g fiber,*
650mg potassium,	*300mg sodium.*

This Spicy Thai Mango and Tofu Salad is a vibrant and heart-healthy dish perfect for a refreshing meal. Firm tofu provides plant-based protein, while mango adds a sweet and tangy flavor rich in vitamins. Mixed salad greens, red bell pepper, and red onion offer a variety of nutrients and a satisfying crunch. Fresh cilantro and mint leaves enhance the salad with their aromatic flavors. The spicy dressing, made with low-sodium soy sauce, rice vinegar, lime juice, sesame oil, and chili flakes, adds a delightful kick. Enjoy this nutritious and delicious salad as a light and flavorful meal.

Roasted Beet and Goat Cheese Salad

Yield: 4 servings | **Prep time:** 15 minutes | **Cook time:** 45 minutes

- **4 medium-sized beets, washed and trimmed**
- **4 cups mixed salad greens (e.g., spinach, arugula, romaine)**
- **1/2 cup crumbled goat cheese**
- **1/4 cup walnuts, toasted**
- **1/4 cup balsamic vinaigrette (homemade or store-bought)**

Nutritional Information:

Approximately 220 calories,	*7g protein,*
20g carbohydrates,	*13g fat,*
15mg cholesterol,	*5g fiber,*
220mg sodium,	

450mg potassium.

1. Preheat the oven to 400°F (200°C). Wrap each beet in aluminum foil and place on a baking sheet. Roast for 45 minutes or until tender when pierced with a fork.
2. Once the beets are cool enough to handle, peel and cut them into bite-sized pieces.
3. In a large salad bowl, combine the mixed greens and roasted beets.
4. Sprinkle the crumbled goat cheese and toasted walnuts over the salad.
5. Drizzle the balsamic vinaigrette over the salad and toss gently to combine all the ingredients.

This Roasted Beet and Goat Cheese Salad is a delightful and heart-healthy dish. Roasted beets provide essential nutrients and antioxidants, supporting cardiovascular health. Mixed salad greens offer a variety of vitamins and minerals, while crumbled goat cheese adds a creamy texture and rich flavor. Toasted walnuts contribute healthy fats and a satisfying crunch. Drizzled with balsamic vinaigrette, this salad is both flavorful and nutritious, making it an excellent choice for a balanced diet. Enjoy this vibrant and delicious salad as a refreshing meal or side dish.

Zucchini Noodle and Pesto Salad

Yield: 4 servings | **Prep time:** 15 minutes | **Cook time:** 0 minutes

- **4 medium zucchinis, spiralized into noodles**
- **1 cup cherry tomatoes, halved**
- **1/4 cup pine nuts, toasted**
- **1 cup homemade or store-bought pesto (preferably low-sodium)**

Nutritional Information:
Approximately 280 calories,
8g protein,
15g carbohydrates,
20g fat,
5g fiber,
10mg cholesterol,
300mg sodium,
680mg potassium.

1. Use a spiralizer to turn the zucchinis into noodles. If you don't have a spiralizer, you can use a vegetable peeler to create long, thin strips.
2. In a large bowl, combine the zucchini noodles and halved cherry tomatoes.
3. Toast the pine nuts in a dry skillet over medium heat for 3–5 minutes, or until golden brown.
4. Add the toasted pine nuts to the zucchini and tomato mixture.
5. Add the pesto to the bowl and toss gently to combine all the ingredients.

This Zucchini Noodle and Pesto Salad is a light, refreshing, and heart-healthy dish perfect for any meal. Spiralized zucchini provides a low-calorie, nutrient-dense base rich in fiber and vitamins. Cherry tomatoes add a burst of flavor and antioxidants, while toasted pine nuts contribute healthy fats and a delightful crunch. The pesto, preferably low-sodium, ties all the ingredients together with its aromatic, savory flavor. This salad is not only delicious but also supports cardiovascular health, making it an excellent choice for a nutritious and satisfying meal.

Green Apple and Walnut Crunch Salad

Yield: 4 servings | **Prep time:** 10 minutes | **Cook time:** 0 minutes

- **2 medium green apples, cored and thinly sliced**
- **1 cup walnuts, roughly chopped**
- **4 cups mixed greens (e.g., spinach, arugula, romaine)**
- **1/2 cup crumbled feta cheese (optional)**
- **1/4 cup balsamic vinaigrette (preferably low-sodium)**

Nutritional Information:
Approximately 250 calories,
7g protein,
20g carbohydrates,
18g fat,
4g fiber,
15mg cholesterol (if using feta),
150mg sodium,
400mg potassium.

1. Core and thinly slice the green apples.
2. In a large bowl, combine the mixed greens, sliced green apples, and chopped walnuts.
3. If using, add the crumbled feta cheese to the bowl.
4. Drizzle the balsamic vinaigrette over the salad ingredients and toss gently to combine.

This Green Apple and Walnut Crunch Salad is a refreshing and heart-healthy dish perfect for any occasion. Green apples provide a crisp texture and a burst of natural sweetness, while walnuts add healthy fats and a satisfying crunch. Mixed greens offer a variety of vitamins and minerals, and optional feta cheese adds a creamy and tangy flavor. The low-sodium balsamic vinaigrette enhances the salad with its tangy sweetness. Enjoy this nutritious and delicious salad as a light meal or a side dish to support cardiovascular health.

Arugula, Orange, and Fennel Salad

Yield: 4 servings | **Prep time:** 15 minutes | **Cook time:** 0 minutes

- **4 cups arugula, washed and dried**
- **2 medium oranges, peeled and segmented**
- **1 medium fennel bulb, thinly sliced**
- **1/4 cup sliced almonds**
- **1/4 cup olive oil**
- **2 tablespoons red wine vinegar**
- **Salt and pepper to taste (use salt sparingly for a heart-healthy option)**

Nutritional Information:

Approximately 200 calories,	*3g protein,*
18g carbohydrates,	*14g fat,*
0mg cholesterol,	*5g fiber,*
400mg potassium,	*50mg sodium.*

1. In a large salad bowl, combine the arugula, orange segments, and thinly sliced fennel.
2. In a separate bowl, whisk together the olive oil and red wine vinegar. Add salt and pepper to taste, if desired.
3. Drizzle the dressing over the salad ingredients and toss gently to combine.
4. Top the salad with sliced almonds before serving.

This Arugula, Orange, and Fennel Salad is a vibrant and heart-healthy dish perfect for a refreshing meal. Arugula provides a peppery base rich in vitamins and antioxidants, while orange segments add a burst of sweetness and vitamin C. Thinly sliced fennel contributes a subtle anise flavor and crunch. Sliced almonds offer healthy fats and a satisfying texture. The simple olive oil and red wine vinegar dressing enhances the flavors without overwhelming them. Enjoy this nutritious salad as a light and delicious addition to your heart-friendly diet.

Grapefruit and Avocado Bliss Salad

Yield: 4 servings | **Prep time:** 15 minutes | **Cook time:** 0 minutes

- **2 large grapefruits, peeled and segmented**
- **2 medium avocados, pitted and sliced**
- **4 cups mixed salad greens (e.g., spinach, arugula, romaine)**
- **1/4 cup chopped walnuts**
- **2 tablespoons olive oil**
- **1 tablespoon lemon juice**
- **Salt and pepper to taste (use salt sparingly for a heart-healthy option)**

Nutritional Information:

Approximately 220 calories,	*4g protein,*
20g carbohydrates,	*16g fat,*
0mg cholesterol,	*6g fiber,*
550mg potassium,	*40mg sodium.*

1. In a large salad bowl, combine the mixed salad greens, grapefruit segments, and avocado slices.
2. In a small bowl, whisk together the olive oil and lemon juice. Add salt and pepper to taste, if desired.
3. Drizzle the dressing over the salad and toss gently to combine.
4. Sprinkle the chopped walnuts on top of the salad before serving.

This Grapefruit and Avocado Bliss Salad is a refreshing and heart-healthy option perfect for any meal. Grapefruit segments provide a tangy sweetness and are rich in vitamin C, while avocado slices offer creamy texture and healthy monounsaturated fats. Mixed salad greens, such as spinach, arugula, and romaine, add a variety of vitamins and antioxidants. Chopped walnuts contribute a satisfying crunch and healthy fats. The olive oil and lemon juice dressing enhances the flavors with a zesty finish. Enjoy this nutritious salad as a light and delicious addition to your heart-friendly diet.

Broccoli and Cranberry Coleslaw

Yield: 4 servings | **Prep time:** 20 minutes | **Cook time:** 0 minutes

- **4 cups broccoli slaw mix (pre-packaged or homemade)**
- **1/2 cup dried cranberries**
- **1/4 cup sunflower seeds**
- **1/4 cup thinly sliced red onion**
- **1/4 cup reduced-fat or light mayonnaise**
- **1 tablespoon apple cider vinegar**
- **1 tablespoon honey or maple syrup (for a vegan option)**
- **Salt and pepper to taste (use salt sparingly for a heart-healthy option)**

Nutritional Information:

Approximately 160 calories,   *4g protein,*

25g carbohydrates,   *6g fat,*

5mg cholesterol,   *4g fiber,*

350mg potassium,   *150mg sodium.*

1. In a large mixing bowl, combine the broccoli slaw mix, dried cranberries, sunflower seeds, and red onion.
2. In a separate small bowl, whisk together the mayonnaise, apple cider vinegar, and honey or maple syrup.
3. Add salt and pepper to taste, if desired. Then, pour the dressing over the slaw mixture.
4. Toss everything together until well combined. Chill in the refrigerator for at least 15 minutes before serving to allow flavors to meld.

This Broccoli and Cranberry Coleslaw is a delicious and heart-healthy side dish perfect for any meal. Broccoli slaw provides a crunchy base rich in fiber and vitamins, supporting cardiovascular health. Dried cranberries add a touch of sweetness and antioxidants, while sunflower seeds contribute healthy fats and protein. Thinly sliced red onion adds a subtle bite. The light mayonnaise dressing, combined with apple cider vinegar and honey or maple syrup, creates a creamy and tangy flavor profile. Enjoy this nutritious coleslaw as a refreshing addition to your heart-friendly diet.

Tomato, Basil, and Mozzarella Caprese

Yield: 4 servings | **Prep time:** 15 minutes | **Cook time:** 0 minutes

- **4 medium tomatoes, sliced into 1/4-inch rounds**
- **1 pound fresh mozzarella cheese, sliced into 1/4-inch rounds**
- **1 bunch fresh basil leaves**
- **1/4 cup extra-virgin olive oil**
- **1 tablespoon balsamic vinegar**
- **Salt and pepper to taste (use salt sparingly for a heart-healthy option)**

Nutritional Information:

Approximately 350 calories,   *20g protein,*

10g carbohydrates,   *28g fat,*

45mg cholesterol,   *2g fiber,*

450mg potassium,   *250mg sodium.*

1. On a large platter, alternately arrange slices of tomato, mozzarella, and basil leaves, creating a circle or overlapping lines.
2. In a small bowl, whisk together extra-virgin olive oil and balsamic vinegar.
3. Drizzle the olive oil and vinegar mixture over the arranged tomato, mozzarella, and basil.
4. Lightly sprinkle salt and pepper to taste, keeping in mind to use salt sparingly for a heart-healthy diet.

This Tomato, Basil, and Mozzarella Caprese is a classic and heart-healthy salad that's both simple and delicious. Fresh tomatoes provide vitamins and antioxidants, while mozzarella offers protein and calcium. Basil leaves add a fragrant touch and a burst of flavor. Drizzled with extra-virgin olive oil and balsamic vinegar, this salad is not only tasty but also rich in healthy fats. Lightly seasoned with salt and pepper, it makes for a refreshing and nutritious dish, perfect for supporting a heart-healthy diet.

Shaved Brussels Sprouts and Parmesan Salad

Yield: 4 servings | Prep time: 15 minutes | Cook time: 0 minutes

- **1 lb Brussels sprouts, shaved or thinly sliced**
- **1/2 cup grated Parmesan cheese (choose a lower-fat option if available)**
- **1/2 cup chopped walnuts**
- **1/4 cup extra-virgin olive oil**
- **Juice of 1 lemon**
- **Salt and pepper to taste (preferably low-sodium salt)**
- **1/2 teaspoon Dijon mustard**

Nutritional Information:

Approximately 280 calories,   *10g protein,*

12g carbohydrates,   *24g fat,*

15mg cholesterol,   *5g fiber,*

450mg potassium,   *280mg sodium.*

1. In a large mixing bowl, combine the shaved Brussels sprouts, grated Parmesan cheese, and chopped walnuts.
2. In a separate small bowl, whisk together the extra-virgin olive oil, lemon juice, salt, pepper, and Dijon mustard to make the dressing.
3. Pour the dressing over the Brussels sprouts mixture and toss to combine.
4. Chill the salad in the refrigerator for about 10 minutes to allow flavors to meld together. Serve chilled.

This Shaved Brussels Sprouts and Parmesan Salad is a nutritious and heart-healthy dish perfect for any meal. Shaved Brussels sprouts provide a crunchy base rich in fiber and vitamins, supporting cardiovascular health. Grated Parmesan cheese adds a savory flavor and protein, while chopped walnuts contribute healthy fats and additional protein. The dressing, made with extra-virgin olive oil, lemon juice, and Dijon mustard, enhances the flavors with a tangy touch. This salad is both delicious and satisfying, making it an excellent choice for a balanced diet. Enjoy it chilled for the best flavor experience.

Sesame-Crusted Tuna and Seaweed Salad

Yield: 4 servings | Prep time: 20 minutes | Cook time: 4 minutes

- **4 fresh tuna steaks (about 5 oz each)**
- **1/4 cup black sesame seeds**
- **1/4 cup white sesame seeds**
- **2 tablespoons low-sodium soy sauce**
- **1 tablespoon olive oil**
- **2 cups seaweed salad (pre-made or homemade)**
- **1 teaspoon wasabi (optional)**
- **1 tablespoon lemon juice**

Nutritional Information:

Approximately 270 calories,

30g protein

8g carbohydrates,

12g fat,

2g fiber,

45mg cholesterol,

300mg sodium,

500mg potassium.

1. Pat the tuna steaks dry with a paper towel. In a shallow dish, mix the black and white sesame seeds together.
2. Dip each tuna steak into the low-sodium soy sauce, coating each side lightly. Then press each side of the tuna into the sesame seed mixture.
3. Heat the olive oil in a non-stick skillet over medium-high heat. Sear the tuna steaks for about 1-2 minutes on each side or until the sesame seeds are golden and fragrant.
4. Slice the tuna steaks thinly and arrange them on top of the seaweed salad. Drizzle with lemon juice and a dab of wasabi if you like it spicy.

This Sesame-Crusted Tuna and Seaweed Salad is a delicious and heart-healthy dish. Fresh tuna steaks are a great source of lean protein and omega-3 fatty acids, promoting cardiovascular health. The sesame seeds add a crunchy texture and healthy fats. Seaweed salad provides additional vitamins, minerals, and antioxidants. Lightly seared and served with a touch of lemon juice and optional wasabi, this dish is flavorful and nutritious. Enjoy this protein-packed meal that supports heart health and overall well-being.

Always remember to add only a minimal amount of salt to the recipe !

Or replace salt with spices on page 10

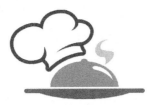

HEART HEALTHY

— ★ ★ ★ ★ ★ —

DIET

Chapter

7

Fish and Seafood

Sesame-Crusted Ahi Tuna Steaks

Yield: 4 servings | **Prep time:** 20 minutes | **Cook time:** 6 minutes

- 4 Ahi Tuna Steaks (about 6 oz each)
- 1/2 cup sesame seeds (white, black, or a mix)
- 2 tablespoons olive oil
- 1/4 cup low-sodium soy sauce
- 1 tablespoon rice vinegar
- 1 teaspoon ginger, grated
- 1 clove garlic, minced
- Salt and pepper to taste
- Optional: Sliced green onions and lemon wedges for garnish

Nutritional Information:

Approximately 340 calories, *40g protein,*
6g carbohydrates, *16g fat,*
60mg cholesterol, *2g fiber,*
450mg potassium, *600mg sodium.*

1. In a shallow dish, mix together soy sauce, rice vinegar, ginger, and garlic. Place the tuna steaks in the marinade and let sit for 10-15 minutes, turning once halfway through.
2. Place sesame seeds on a plate. Remove tuna from marinade and season with a pinch of salt and pepper. Press each side of the tuna steaks into the sesame seeds to form a crust.
3. Heat olive oil in a non-stick skillet over medium-high heat. Once hot, add the tuna steaks.
4. Cook for 2-3 minutes on each side for medium-rare, adjusting the time for your desired level of doneness.
5. Remove from heat, let rest for a few minutes and then slice. Garnish with optional green onions and lemon wedges if desired.

These Sesame-Crusted Ahi Tuna Steaks are a flavorful and heart-healthy dish. Ahi tuna provides lean protein and omega-3 fatty acids, essential for cardiovascular health. The sesame seeds create a crunchy crust, adding a nutty flavor and healthy fats. Marinated in a mixture of low-sodium soy sauce, rice vinegar, ginger, and garlic, the tuna steaks are packed with flavor. Quick to prepare and cook, this dish is perfect for a nutritious meal. Garnish with sliced green onions and lemon wedges for an extra touch of freshness and enjoy this delicious, healthy recipe.

Lemon-Herb Grilled Salmon

Yield: 4 servings | **Prep time:** 15 minutes | **Cook time:** 10 minutes

- **4 salmon fillets, 6 ounces each**
- **Zest and juice of 1 lemon**
- **2 tablespoons olive oil**
- **2 cloves garlic, minced**
- **1 teaspoon dried oregano**
- **1 teaspoon dried thyme**
- **Salt and pepper to taste**
- **Fresh parsley for garnish (optional)**

Nutritional Information:

Approximately 340 calories,	*34g protein,*
3g carbohydrates,	*21g fat,*
95mg cholesterol,	*0g fiber,*
850mg potassium,	*150mg sodium.*

1. In a small bowl, whisk together lemon zest, lemon juice, olive oil, garlic, oregano, thyme, salt, and pepper.
2. Place the salmon fillets in a shallow dish and pour the marinade over them. Cover and let marinate in the refrigerator for at least 10 minutes, up to 30 minutes.
3. Preheat the grill to medium-high heat. Remove the salmon from the marinade and discard the marinade.
4. Place the salmon fillets skin-side down on the grill. Grill for about 4-5 minutes per side, or until the salmon flakes easily with a fork.
5. Serve immediately, garnished with fresh parsley if desired.

This Lemon-Herb Grilled Salmon is a flavorful and heart-healthy dish perfect for a nutritious meal. Salmon fillets provide a rich source of omega-3 fatty acids and high-quality protein, which are essential for cardiovascular health. The lemon zest and juice add a bright, tangy flavor, while olive oil, garlic, oregano, and thyme enhance the dish with aromatic herbs. Grilled to perfection, this salmon is both delicious and nutritious. Garnish with fresh parsley for an extra touch of freshness. Enjoy this easy and healthy recipe as part of a balanced diet.

Spiced Tilapia Tacos with Avocado Crema

Yield: 4 servings | **Prep time:** 20 minutes | **Cook time:** 10 minutes

For the Tilapia:
- **4 tilapia fillets (about 4-5 ounces each)**
- **1 tablespoon olive oil**
- **1 teaspoon ground cumin**
- **1 teaspoon paprika**
- **1/2 teaspoon garlic powder**
- **Salt and pepper to taste**

For the Avocado Crema:
- **1 ripe avocado, peeled and pitted**
- **1/2 cup plain Greek yogurt**
- **Juice of 1 lime**
- **Salt to taste**

For assembling:
- **8 small whole-grain corn tortillas**
- **1 cup shredded lettuce**
- **1/2 cup diced tomatoes**
- **1/4 cup diced red onion**

1. Preheat the oven to 400°F (200°C). Place the tilapia fillets on a baking sheet lined with parchment paper. Drizzle olive oil over the fillets and sprinkle with cumin, paprika, garlic powder, salt, and pepper. Bake for 10 minutes or until the fish flakes easily with a fork.
2. While the fish is baking, prepare the avocado crema by blending avocado, Greek yogurt, lime juice, and salt in a blender until smooth.
3. Warm the tortillas according to package directions.
4. Assemble the tacos by placing a portion of the cooked tilapia on a tortilla, followed by avocado crema, shredded lettuce, diced tomatoes, and red onion.
5. Serve immediately.

Nutritional Information:

Approximately 410 calories,	*30g protein,*
32g carbohydrates,	*18g fat,*
55mg cholesterol,	*8g fiber,*
700mg potassium,	*350mg sodium.*

These Spiced Tilapia Tacos with Avocado Crema are a flavorful and heart-healthy meal. Tilapia fillets are seasoned with cumin, paprika, and garlic powder, then baked to perfection. The creamy avocado crema, made with ripe avocado, Greek yogurt, and lime juice, adds a refreshing contrast. Whole-grain corn tortillas provide a fiber-rich base, and the toppings of shredded lettuce, diced tomatoes, and red onion add crunch and nutrients. This dish is delicious, nutritious, and perfect for a balanced diet. Enjoy these tacos for a satisfying and heart-friendly meal.

Baked Cod with Mediterranean Salsa

Yield: 4 servings | **Prep time:** 15 minutes | **Cook time:** 15 minutes

For the Cod:
- **4 cod fillets (about 6 ounces each)**
- **1 tablespoon olive oil**
- **Salt and pepper to taste**

For the Mediterranean Salsa:
- **1 cup cherry tomatoes, halved**
- **1/2 cup cucumber, diced**
- **1/4 cup red onion, finely chopped**
- **1/4 cup Kalamata olives, pitted and sliced**
- **2 tablespoons capers, drained**
- **1 tablespoon olive oil**
- **Juice of 1 lemon**
- **2 tablespoons fresh parsley, chopped**
- **Salt and pepper to taste**

1. Preheat the oven to 400°F (200°C). Line a baking sheet with parchment paper.
2. Place the cod fillets on the prepared baking sheet, drizzle with olive oil, and season with salt and pepper. Bake for 12-15 minutes or until the fish flakes easily with a fork.
3. While the fish is baking, prepare the Mediterranean salsa by combining cherry tomatoes, cucumber, red onion, olives, capers, olive oil, lemon juice, and parsley in a bowl. Season with salt and pepper to taste.
4. Once the fish is done, carefully remove it from the oven. Serve each fillet topped with a generous spoonful of Mediterranean salsa.

Nutritional Information:

Approximately 250 calories, *30g protein,*
8g carbohydrates, *11g fat,*
60mg cholesterol, *2g fiber,*
600mg potassium, *400mg sodium.*

This Baked Cod with Mediterranean Salsa is a light and heart-healthy dish perfect for a nutritious meal. Cod fillets are baked to perfection, providing a lean source of protein and omega-3 fatty acids. The Mediterranean salsa, made with cherry tomatoes, cucumber, red onion, Kalamata olives, capers, and fresh parsley, adds a burst of flavor and antioxidants. Drizzled with olive oil and lemon juice, this dish is both delicious and nutritious. Enjoy this easy-to-make recipe for a balanced and satisfying meal that supports cardiovascular health.

Garlic and Rosemary Sea Bass

Yield: 4 servings | **Prep time:** 10 minutes | **Cook time:** 12 minutes

- **4 sea bass fillets (about 6 ounces each)**
- **3 tablespoons olive oil**
- **4 garlic cloves, minced**
- **2 tablespoons fresh rosemary, finely chopped**
- **Zest and juice of 1 lemon**
- **Salt and pepper to taste**

1. Preheat the oven to 400°F (200°C). Line a baking sheet with parchment paper or lightly grease it.
2. In a small bowl, mix together the olive oil, minced garlic, rosemary, lemon zest, and lemon juice.
3. Place the sea bass fillets skin-side down on the prepared baking sheet. Season them with salt and pepper to taste.
4. Generously brush the olive oil mixture over the fillets.
5. Bake for 10-12 minutes or until the fish flakes easily with a fork.

Nutritional Information:

Approximately 270 calories, *34g protein,*
1g carbohydrates, *14g fat,*
75mg cholesterol, *0g fiber,*
400mg potassium, *100mg sodium.*

This Garlic and Rosemary Sea Bass is a flavorful and heart-healthy dish perfect for any meal. Sea bass fillets provide a lean source of protein and omega-3 fatty acids, which support cardiovascular health. The olive oil mixture with minced garlic, fresh rosemary, lemon zest, and lemon juice adds a delightful aroma and tangy flavor. Baked to perfection, this sea bass is both delicious and nutritious. Enjoy this easy-to-make recipe as a light and satisfying meal, ideal for a balanced and heart-friendly diet.

Shrimp and Asparagus Stir-Fry

Yield: 4 servings | **Prep time:** 15 minutes | **Cook time:** 10 minutes

- 1 pound large shrimp, peeled and deveined
- 1 bunch asparagus, trimmed and cut into 2-inch pieces (about 1 pound)
- 2 tablespoons olive oil
- 4 garlic cloves, minced
- 1 teaspoon ginger, grated
- 2 tablespoons low-sodium soy sauce
- 1 tablespoon oyster sauce (optional)
- Zest and juice of 1 lemon
- Salt and pepper to taste
- 1 tablespoon sesame seeds (for garnish, optional)

Nutritional Information:

Approximately 220 calories,	25g protein,
8g carbohydrates,	10g fat,
180mg cholesterol,	3g fiber,
400mg potassium,	420mg sodium.

1. In a large skillet or wok, heat the olive oil over medium-high heat. Add the garlic and ginger, sautéing for about 30 seconds until fragrant.
2. Add the asparagus to the skillet and stir-fry for about 4-5 minutes, or until they start to become tender.
3. Add the shrimp to the skillet along with the soy sauce, oyster sauce (if using), lemon zest, and lemon juice. Stir to combine.
4. Cook for another 4-5 minutes, or until the shrimp are pink and cooked through. Season with salt and pepper to taste.
5. Garnish with sesame seeds before serving, if desired.

This Shrimp and Asparagus Stir-Fry is a quick, delicious, and heart-healthy meal. Shrimp provides a lean source of protein and essential omega-3 fatty acids, while asparagus is rich in vitamins and fiber. The combination of garlic, ginger, and lemon zest adds a fresh and aromatic flavor. Low-sodium soy sauce and optional oyster sauce enhance the taste without adding excess sodium. This stir-fry is easy to prepare and perfect for a nutritious dinner. Garnish with sesame seeds for added texture and enjoy this flavorful dish that supports cardiovascular health.

Poached Halibut in White Wine Broth

Yield: 4 servings | **Prep time:** 15 minutes | **Cook time:** 15 minutes

- 4 Halibut fillets (about 6 oz each)
- 1 cup dry white wine
- 1 cup low-sodium vegetable broth
- 1 onion, thinly sliced
- 2 cloves garlic, minced
- 2 tablespoons olive oil
- 1 lemon, sliced
- Fresh herbs such as thyme and parsley for garnish
- Salt and pepper to taste

Nutritional Information:

Approximately 320 calories,	36g protein,
8g carbohydrates,	12g fat,
55mg cholesterol,	1g fiber,
650mg potassium,	270mg sodium.

1. In a large skillet, heat olive oil over medium heat. Add sliced onion and minced garlic, and sauté until softened, about 3-5 minutes.
2. Pour in the white wine and vegetable broth, then bring the mixture to a simmer.
3. Season the halibut fillets with salt and pepper, and gently place them in the simmering broth. Add lemon slices on top.
4. Cover the skillet and simmer for about 8-10 minutes, or until the fish is cooked through and flakes easily.
5. Serve immediately, garnished with fresh herbs like thyme and parsley.

This Poached Halibut in White Wine Broth is a delicate and heart-healthy dish perfect for a sophisticated meal. Halibut fillets provide a lean source of protein and essential nutrients. The poaching liquid, made from dry white wine and low-sodium vegetable broth, imparts a rich and savory flavor without adding excess calories or sodium. Sautéed onion and garlic add depth, while lemon slices and fresh herbs like thyme and parsley enhance the dish with fresh, aromatic notes. Enjoy this elegant and nutritious meal as part of a balanced diet.

Coconut-Curry Mussels

Yield: 4 servings | **Prep time:** 15 minutes | **Cook time:** 10 minutes

- **2 pounds fresh mussels, scrubbed and de-bearded**
- **1 can (14 oz) light coconut milk**
- **1 tablespoon olive oil**
- **1 small onion, finely chopped**
- **2 cloves garlic, minced**
- **1 tablespoon fresh ginger, grated**
- **1 tablespoon curry powder**
- **1 lime, juiced**
- **Salt to taste**
- **Fresh cilantro leaves for garnish**

Nutritional Information:

Approximately 290 calories,	*22g protein,*
16g carbohydrates,	*14g fat,*
48mg cholesterol,	*2g fiber,*
640mg potassium,	*550mg sodium.*

1. Heat olive oil in a large pot over medium heat. Add the chopped onion, garlic, and ginger, sautéing until the onion becomes translucent, about 3 minutes.
2. Stir in the curry powder and cook for an additional 1 minute, allowing the flavors to meld.
3. Pour in the light coconut milk and bring the mixture to a simmer.
4. Add the scrubbed mussels to the pot, cover, and cook for about 5-7 minutes or until the mussels have opened. Discard any mussels that do not open.
5. Stir in the lime juice and season with salt to taste. Serve immediately, garnished with fresh cilantro leaves.

These Coconut-Curry Mussels are a flavorful and heart-healthy dish perfect for a special meal. Fresh mussels provide lean protein and essential minerals. The rich and aromatic broth, made with light coconut milk, curry powder, and fresh ginger, enhances the natural flavor of the mussels. Onion, garlic, and lime juice add depth and brightness to the dish, while fresh cilantro offers a burst of freshness. This quick and easy recipe is both delicious and nutritious, making it an excellent choice for a balanced and heart-friendly diet.

Grilled Swordfish with Pineapple Salsa

Yield: 4 servings | **Prep time:** 25 minutes | **Cook time:** 10 minutes

- **4 swordfish steaks (about 6 oz each)**
- **1 tablespoon olive oil**
- **Salt and pepper to taste**
- **2 cups fresh pineapple, diced**
- **1 small red onion, finely chopped**
- **1 jalapeño, seeded and finely chopped**
- **1/4 cup fresh cilantro, chopped**
- **Juice of 1 lime**
- **1 teaspoon honey (optional)**

Nutritional Information:

Approximately 270 calories,	*28g protein,*
15g carbohydrates,	*10g fat,*
55mg cholesterol,	*2g fiber,*
520mg potassium,	*210mg sodium.*

1. Preheat the grill to medium-high heat. Rub the swordfish steaks with olive oil and season with salt and pepper. Set aside to marinate while you prepare the salsa.
2. In a bowl, combine the diced pineapple, red onion, jalapeño, cilantro, lime juice, and honey (if using). Stir well to combine and set aside.
3. Place the swordfish steaks on the preheated grill and cook for about 4-5 minutes per side, or until the fish is opaque and flakes easily.
4. Remove the swordfish from the grill and serve immediately, topped with a generous spoonful of pineapple salsa.

This Grilled Swordfish with Pineapple Salsa is a delightful and heart-healthy dish perfect for a flavorful meal. Swordfish steaks provide a lean source of protein and essential nutrients. The vibrant pineapple salsa, made with fresh pineapple, red onion, jalapeño, cilantro, and lime juice, adds a refreshing and tangy contrast to the rich fish. Grilling the swordfish enhances its natural flavors, making it a delicious and nutritious option. Enjoy this easy-to-make recipe for a balanced and heart-friendly meal that is sure to impress.

Pan-Seared Trout with Almond Butter

Yield: 4 servings | **Prep time:** 10 minutes | **Cook time:** 12 minutes

- **4 trout fillets (about 6 oz each)**
- **1 tablespoon olive oil**
- **Salt and pepper to taste**
- **1/4 cup almond butter**
- **Juice of 1 lemon**
- **1 garlic clove, minced**
- **1 tablespoon fresh parsley, chopped**
- **1/4 cup slivered almonds, toasted**

Nutritional Information:

Approximately 350 calories,   *32g protein,*

8g carbohydrates,   *22g fat,*

85mg cholesterol,   *3g fiber,*

620mg potassium,   *170mg sodium.*

1. Preheat a non-stick skillet over medium heat and add the olive oil.
2. Season the trout fillets with salt and pepper. Place the fillets skin-side down in the skillet and cook for 5-6 minutes per side, or until the fish is cooked through and flakes easily with a fork.
3. In a small bowl, mix together the almond butter, lemon juice, minced garlic, and parsley. Warm the mixture in the microwave for about 20-30 seconds, stirring well.
4. To serve, place each trout fillet on a plate and spoon a generous amount of almond butter sauce over the top. Sprinkle with toasted slivered almonds.

This Pan-Seared Trout with Almond Butter is a delicious and heart-healthy dish perfect for a nutritious meal. Trout fillets provide a lean source of protein and essential omega-3 fatty acids, which are beneficial for heart health. The almond butter sauce, infused with lemon juice, garlic, and parsley, adds a rich and nutty flavor, enhancing the trout's natural taste. Toasted slivered almonds add a delightful crunch, making this dish both flavorful and satisfying. Enjoy this easy and elegant recipe as part of a balanced and heart-friendly diet.

Roasted Red Snapper with Fennel and Olives

Yield: 4 servings | **Prep time:** 15 minutes | **Cook time:** 20 minutes

- **4 red snapper fillets (about 6 oz each)**
- **1 large fennel bulb, thinly sliced**
- **1 cup cherry tomatoes, halved**
- **1/2 cup pitted Kalamata olives**
- **2 tablespoons olive oil**
- **Zest and juice of 1 lemon**
- **Salt and pepper to taste**
- **2 cloves garlic, minced**
- **1 teaspoon dried oregano**
- **2 tablespoons chopped fresh parsley for garnish**

Nutritional Information:

Approximately 275 calories,   *35g protein,*

9g carbohydrates,   *11g fat,*

50mg cholesterol,   *3g fiber,*

700mg potassium,   *300mg sodium*

1. Preheat your oven to 400°F (200°C). In a large baking dish, spread the thinly sliced fennel, cherry tomatoes, and Kalamata olives.
2. In a small bowl, mix the olive oil, lemon zest, lemon juice, garlic, dried oregano, salt, and pepper. Drizzle this mixture over the fennel and tomatoes in the baking dish.
3. Place the red snapper fillets on top of the fennel and tomatoes. Season the fillets with additional salt and pepper if desired.
4. Roast in the preheated oven for 18-20 minutes, or until the fish flakes easily with a fork and the fennel is tender.
5. Garnish with chopped fresh parsley before serving.

Enjoy a flavorful and healthy meal with this Roasted Red Snapper with Fennel and Olives recipe. This dish combines the delicate taste of red snapper with the aromatic flavors of fennel, cherry tomatoes, and Kalamata olives, all roasted to perfection. The addition of lemon zest, garlic, and dried oregano enhances the dish, making it a delightful and nutritious option for a balanced diet. Garnished with fresh parsley, this meal is as visually appealing as it is delicious, perfect for a heart-healthy lifestyle.

Blackened Mahi-Mahi with Mango-Avocado Relish

Yield: 4 servings | **Prep time:** 20 minutes | **Cook time:** 10 minutes

For the Mahi-Mahi:
- **4 Mahi-Mahi fillets (about 6 oz each)**
- **1 tablespoon olive oil**
- **2 teaspoons paprika**
- **1 teaspoon garlic powder**
- **1 teaspoon onion powder**
- **1/2 teaspoon cayenne pepper**
- **1/2 teaspoon black pepper**
- **1/2 teaspoon salt**

For the Mango-Avocado Relish:
- **1 ripe mango, diced**
- **1 ripe avocado, diced**
- **1/4 cup red onion, finely chopped**
- **Juice of 1 lime**
- **2 tablespoons chopped cilantro**
- **Salt to taste**

1. In a small bowl, combine paprika, garlic powder, onion powder, cayenne pepper, black pepper, and salt. Rub this spice mix generously on both sides of each Mahi-Mahi fillet.
2. Heat olive oil in a non-stick skillet over medium-high heat. Add the Mahi-Mahi fillets and cook for 4-5 minutes on each side, or until fish is cooked through and has a nice blackened crust.
3. While the fish is cooking, prepare the Mango-Avocado Relish. In a medium bowl, combine diced mango, avocado, red onion, lime juice, cilantro, and salt. Toss gently to combine.
4. Serve the blackened Mahi-Mahi hot, topped with Mango-Avocado Relish.

Nutritional Information:
Approximately 320 calories, 20g carbohydrates, 120mg cholesterol, 750mg potassium, 35g protein, 12g fat, 5g fiber, 420mg sodium.

Blackened Mahi-Mahi with Mango-Avocado Relish is a heart-healthy recipe perfect for those following a diet for cardiovascular wellness. Mahi-Mahi is a lean fish rich in omega-3 fatty acids, which are known to support heart health by reducing inflammation and lowering blood pressure. The mango-avocado relish adds a fresh, vibrant flavor while providing essential vitamins, healthy fats, and fiber. This dish is low in sodium and high in potassium, making it an excellent choice for maintaining healthy blood pressure levels. Enjoy this delicious, nutritious meal that supports your heart health goals.

Spicy Shrimp Ceviche

Yield: 4 servings | **Prep time:** 25 minutes | **Cook time:** 0 minutes (Ceviche is not cooked)

- **1 pound large shrimp, peeled, deveined, and diced**
- **Juice of 3 limes**
- **Juice of 1 lemon**
- **1 small red onion, finely chopped**
- **1 jalapeño, seeds removed and finely chopped**
- **1 medium tomato, diced**
- **1/2 cup chopped cilantro**
- **1 avocado, diced**
- **Salt and pepper to taste**

1. In a medium glass bowl, combine shrimp and the juices of the limes and lemon. Make sure the shrimp is well covered with the juice. Cover and refrigerate for about 20 minutes, or until shrimp turns pink and opaque.
2. Drain off excess citrus juice, leaving just enough to keep the mixture moist.
3. Add red onion, jalapeño, tomato, and cilantro to the shrimp. Stir until well mixed.
4. Gently fold in diced avocado, and season with salt and pepper to taste.
5. Serve immediately with tortilla chips or over a bed of lettuce, or refrigerate until ready to serve.

Nutritional Information:
Approximately 220 calories, 12g carbohydrates, 180mg cholesterol, 700mg potassium, 25g protein, 8g fat, 5g fiber, 400mg sodium.

Spicy Shrimp Ceviche is a refreshing and heart-healthy dish perfect for a diet focused on cardiovascular wellness. Shrimp is a lean source of protein and low in saturated fat, promoting healthy cholesterol levels. The ceviche is packed with fresh vegetables like tomatoes and avocados, which provide essential vitamins, minerals, and fiber to support heart health. The lime and lemon juice not only add a zesty flavor but also supply a dose of vitamin C. This vibrant dish is low in calories and sodium, making it an excellent choice for a nutritious, heart-friendly meal.

Honey-Mustard Glazed Salmon

Yield: 4 servings | **Prep time:** 10 minutes | **Cook time:** 15 minutes

- **4 (6-ounce) salmon fillets**
- **2 tablespoons honey**
- **2 tablespoons Dijon mustard**
- **1 tablespoon olive oil**
- **1 teaspoon minced garlic**
- **Salt and pepper to taste**
- **1 lemon, thinly sliced for garnish (optional)**
- **1 tablespoon chopped fresh parsley for garnish (optional)**

Nutritional Information:

Approximately 340 calories,	*35g protein,*
18g carbohydrates,	*14g fat,*
90mg cholesterol,	*0g fiber,*
650mg potassium,	*350mg sodium.*

1. Preheat your oven to 400°F (200°C). Line a baking sheet with parchment paper or lightly grease it.
2. In a small bowl, whisk together honey, Dijon mustard, olive oil, and minced garlic.
3. Place the salmon fillets on the prepared baking sheet, skin-side down. Season with salt and pepper.
4. Generously brush the honey-mustard mixture over the salmon fillets.
5. Bake in the preheated oven for 12-15 minutes, or until the salmon flakes easily with a fork. Garnish with lemon slices and chopped parsley if desired.

Honey-Mustard Glazed Salmon is an excellent choice for a heart-healthy diet, rich in omega-3 fatty acids that support cardiovascular health by reducing inflammation and lowering blood pressure. The glaze made with honey and Dijon mustard adds a delightful flavor without the need for excessive salt or unhealthy fats. Salmon is also high in protein and provides essential vitamins and minerals, making it a nutritious and satisfying meal. This easy-to-prepare dish combines taste and nutrition, promoting heart health and overall wellness with every bite.

Asian-Style Steamed Clams

Yield: 4 servings | **Prep time:** 15 minutes | **Cook time:** 10 minutes

- **2 lbs fresh clams, cleaned and purged**
- **1 cup low-sodium chicken or vegetable broth**
- **1/2 cup white wine (optional)**
- **3 cloves garlic, minced**
- **1-inch ginger root, thinly sliced**
- **1/4 cup low-sodium soy sauce**
- **1 tablespoon sesame oil**
- **2 green onions, chopped**
- **1 small red chili, thinly sliced (optional)**
- **A handful of fresh cilantro leaves for garnish**

Nutritional Information:

Approximately 190 calories,	*22g protein,*
9g carbohydrates,	*4g fat,*
50mg cholesterol,	*0g fiber,*
520mg potassium,	*450mg sodium.*

1. In a large pot, combine the broth, white wine (if using), minced garlic, and ginger slices. Bring the liquid to a simmer over medium heat.
2. Add the cleaned clams to the pot, cover, and steam for 7-10 minutes or until all the clams have opened. Discard any clams that do not open.
3. In a small bowl, mix together the low-sodium soy sauce and sesame oil.
4. Once the clams are cooked, drizzle the soy sauce and sesame oil mixture over them. Toss to combine.
5. Garnish with chopped green onions, red chili slices (if using), and fresh cilantro leaves. Serve immediately.

Asian-Style Steamed Clams are a flavorful and heart-healthy seafood dish ideal for a diet focused on cardiovascular wellness. Clams are a rich source of lean protein and essential nutrients, while low-sodium soy sauce and sesame oil add depth of flavor without excess sodium, supporting heart health. The addition of garlic and ginger not only enhances the dish with aromatic notes but also provides anti-inflammatory and antioxidant benefits. Topped with fresh cilantro and a hint of chili, this dish is both vibrant and nutritious, perfect for a wholesome meal.

Walnut-Crusted Flounder with Spinach

Yield: 4 servings | **Prep time:** 20 minutes | **Cook time:** 15 minutes

- 4 flounder fillets (about 4 oz each)
- 1 cup walnuts, finely chopped
- 1 tablespoon olive oil
- Salt and pepper to taste
- 1 egg, beaten
- 4 cups fresh spinach leaves
- 2 cloves garlic, minced
- 1 lemon, cut into wedges

Nutritional Information:

Approximately 320 calories,	*28g protein,*
6g carbohydrates,	*21g fat,*
85mg cholesterol,	*3g fiber,*
550mg potassium,	*250mg sodium.*

1. Preheat your oven to 400°F (200°C). Line a baking sheet with parchment paper.
2. In a shallow dish, place the beaten egg. In another dish, place the finely chopped walnuts. Dip each flounder fillet into the egg, then press it into the walnuts, making sure the fillet is well coated.
3. Place the walnut-crusted fillets on the prepared baking sheet, drizzle with a tablespoon of olive oil, and season with salt and pepper. Bake for 12-15 minutes, or until the fish flakes easily with a fork.
4. While the fish is baking, heat a large skillet over medium heat. Add the garlic and sauté for 1 minute. Add the spinach and cook until wilted, about 3-4 minutes.
5. Serve the walnut-crusted flounder over a bed of sautéed spinach and garnish with lemon wedges.

Walnut-Crusted Flounder with Spinach is an excellent choice for a heart-healthy diet. The flounder provides lean protein and essential omega-3 fatty acids, which are beneficial for heart health. Walnuts add a crunchy texture and are rich in heart-healthy fats, antioxidants, and anti-inflammatory properties. The bed of fresh spinach not only enhances the dish's flavor but also contributes iron, vitamins, and fiber, promoting overall cardiovascular wellness. This recipe combines nutritious ingredients into a delicious meal, perfect for maintaining a healthy heart.

Herb-Stuffed Whole Rainbow Trout

Yield: 4 servings | **Prep time:** 20 minutes | **Cook time:** 25 minutes

- 4 whole rainbow trout, cleaned and gutted (about 1-1.5 pounds each)
- 1 tablespoon olive oil
- 2 cloves garlic, minced
- 1 lemon, thinly sliced
- 1/2 cup fresh herbs (parsley, dill, thyme), chopped
- Salt and pepper to taste
- 1/4 cup white wine (optional)

Nutritional Information:

Approximately 310 calories,	*45g protein,*
2g carbohydrates,	*12g fat,*
100mg cholesterol,	*0g fiber,*
600mg potassium.	*180mg sodium,*

1. Preheat your oven to 375°F (190°C). Lightly oil a large baking sheet.
2. In a small bowl, mix together the minced garlic, chopped herbs, salt, and pepper.
3. Open up each cleaned rainbow trout like a book, and rub the inside with a little olive oil. Then stuff with the herb mixture and a few lemon slices.
4. Place the stuffed trout on the baking sheet and drizzle with white wine if using. Bake for 20-25 minutes, or until the fish flakes easily when tested with a fork.
5. Serve hot, garnished with additional lemon slices and herbs if desired.

Herb-Stuffed Whole Rainbow Trout is a delightful dish packed with flavor and health benefits, making it an excellent choice for a heart-healthy diet. Rainbow trout is rich in omega-3 fatty acids, which are known to reduce inflammation and improve heart health. The fresh herbs and garlic add antioxidants and anti-inflammatory properties, while the use of olive oil provides healthy monounsaturated fats. This simple yet elegant dish is low in carbohydrates and high in protein, making it a nutritious meal option that supports cardiovascular wellness.

Barramundi in Lemon-Caper Sauce

Yield: 4 servings | **Prep time:** 10 minutes | **Cook time:** 12 minutes

- 4 barramundi fillets (about 6 oz each)
- 2 tablespoons olive oil
- Salt and pepper to taste
- 1 lemon, juiced and zested
- 2 tablespoons capers, drained
- 1/4 cup low-sodium chicken or vegetable broth
- 1 tablespoon fresh parsley, finely chopped
- 1 garlic clove, minced

Nutritional Information:

Approximately 220 calories,	27g protein,
4g carbohydrates,	11g fat,
60mg cholesterol,	1g fiber,
600mg potassium,	300mg sodium.

1. Season the barramundi fillets with salt and pepper. Heat olive oil in a large skillet over medium-high heat. Add the fillets and cook for about 4 minutes per side or until they easily flake with a fork. Remove the fillets and set them aside.
2. In the same skillet, add minced garlic and sauté for about 1 minute until fragrant. Add the lemon juice, lemon zest, capers, and broth. Bring to a simmer and cook for 3 minutes to reduce slightly.
3. Return the barramundi fillets to the skillet and spoon some of the sauce over them. Simmer for another 2 minutes to allow the flavors to combine.
4. Transfer the fillets to a serving plate, spoon the sauce over the top, and garnish with chopped parsley.
5. Serve immediately, optionally with a side of steamed vegetables or whole-grain rice.

Barramundi in Lemon-Caper Sauce is a delightful dish perfect for a heart-healthy diet. Barramundi is a lean source of protein rich in omega-3 fatty acids, which help reduce inflammation and improve heart health. The lemon-caper sauce adds a zesty flavor without adding extra calories or unhealthy fats. Capers provide antioxidants and a unique taste, while the use of olive oil ensures a dose of heart-healthy monounsaturated fats. This recipe offers a balanced, flavorful meal that supports cardiovascular wellness.

Lobster Salad with Baby Greens

Yield: 4 servings | **Prep time:** 25 minutes | **Cook time:** 10 minutes

- 1 pound cooked lobster meat, cut into bite-sized pieces
- 6 cups mixed baby greens (e.g., spinach, arugula, kale)
- 1 medium avocado, diced
- 1/2 cup cherry tomatoes, halved
- 1/4 cup red onion, thinly sliced
- 2 tablespoons olive oil
- 1 tablespoon lemon juice
- Salt and pepper to taste

Nutritional Information:

Approximately 280 calories,	22g protein,
10g carbohydrates,	16g fat,
60mg cholesterol,	4g fiber,
600mg potassium,	300mg sodium.

1. In a large bowl, combine the mixed baby greens, diced avocado, cherry tomatoes, and thinly sliced red onion.
2. In a small bowl, whisk together the olive oil, lemon juice, salt, and pepper to make the dressing.
3. Add the cooked lobster meat to the large bowl with the greens and other veggies.
4. Drizzle the dressing over the salad and toss gently to combine all ingredients evenly.
5. Divide the salad among four plates and serve immediately.

Lobster Salad with Baby Greens is a luxurious yet heart-healthy option, perfect for a light meal. Lobster is an excellent source of lean protein, which helps maintain muscle mass and supports overall health. Combined with nutrient-dense baby greens like spinach, arugula, and kale, this salad offers a rich supply of vitamins, minerals, and antioxidants that promote heart health. Avocado adds healthy monounsaturated fats, which can help lower bad cholesterol levels, while the light lemon-olive oil dressing enhances the flavors without adding unhealthy fats. This salad is a delicious way to enjoy a nutritious, heart-healthy meal.

Saffron-Infused Seafood Paella

Yield: 6 servings | **Prep time:** 20 minutes | **Cook time:** 40 minutes

- **1 tablespoon olive oil**
- **1 medium onion, finely chopped**
- **2 cloves garlic, minced**
- **1 red bell pepper, diced**
- **1 1/2 cups short-grain brown rice**
- **1/4 teaspoon saffron threads**
- **4 cups low-sodium vegetable broth**
- **1 pound mixed seafood (shrimp, mussels, and calamari), cleaned and shells removed from shrimp**
- **1 cup diced tomatoes (canned or fresh)**
- **1 cup frozen peas, thawed**
- **1 lemon, cut into wedges**
- **Salt and pepper to taste**
- **Fresh parsley for garnish**

Nutritional Information:

Approximately 350 calories, 28g protein, 50g carbohydrates, 5g fat, 80mg cholesterol, 6g fiber, 400mg potassium, 500mg sodium.

1. In a large paella pan or wide skillet, heat the olive oil over medium heat. Add the onion, garlic, and red bell pepper. Sauté until softened, about 5 minutes.
2. Add the rice and saffron threads to the skillet. Stir to coat the rice in the saffron and oil. Cook for 2-3 minutes, allowing the rice to slightly toast.
3. Pour in the vegetable broth and bring to a simmer. Cover and cook for about 25 minutes, or until the rice is nearly cooked through.
4. Stir in the mixed seafood, diced tomatoes, and peas. Cover and cook for an additional 10 minutes, or until the seafood is cooked through.
5. Serve the paella hot, garnished with lemon wedges and fresh parsley.

Saffron-Infused Seafood Paella is a flavorful and nutritious dish that perfectly aligns with a heart-healthy diet. The combination of mixed seafood such as shrimp, mussels, and calamari provides lean protein and omega-3 fatty acids, which are beneficial for cardiovascular health. Saffron adds a unique flavor and vibrant color while also offering antioxidant properties. Using short-grain brown rice increases fiber content, aiding in cholesterol management. This paella is low in fat and sodium, making it a delicious and wholesome meal option for maintaining a healthy heart.

Miso-Glazed Scallops

Yield: 4 servings | **Prep time:** 15 minutes | **Cook time:** 8 minutes

- **1.5 pounds sea scallops (about 16)**
- **1/4 cup white miso paste**
- **2 tablespoons low-sodium soy sauce**
- **1 tablespoon mirin (sweet rice wine)**
- **1 tablespoon rice vinegar**
- **2 teaspoons sesame oil**
- **1 teaspoon honey**
- **2 green onions, finely chopped for garnish**
- **1 tablespoon olive oil for searing**

Nutritional Information:

Approximately 230 calories, 25g protein, 14g carbohydrates, 8g fat, 45mg cholesterol, 1g fiber, 500mg potassium, 600mg sodium.

1. In a small bowl, whisk together the miso paste, low-sodium soy sauce, mirin, rice vinegar, sesame oil, and honey to make the glaze.
2. In a large bowl, toss the scallops with half of the miso glaze, making sure they are evenly coated. Let them marinate for about 10 minutes.
3. Heat the olive oil in a large skillet over medium-high heat. Once hot, add the scallops and cook for 3-4 minutes per side, or until they are opaque and slightly browned.
4. Drizzle the remaining miso glaze over the cooked scallops and garnish with chopped green onions.

Miso-Glazed Scallops offer a deliciously savory and heart-healthy option for seafood lovers. Scallops are low in fat and high in protein, making them an excellent choice for maintaining muscle mass and supporting overall heart health. The miso glaze, made with white miso paste, low-sodium soy sauce, mirin, rice vinegar, and honey, adds a burst of umami flavor without excessive sodium. Sesame oil provides healthy fats, and green onions add a fresh, nutritious garnish. This dish is both flavorful and nutritious, making it a perfect addition to a heart-healthy diet.

HEART HEALTHY

— ★★★★★ —

DIET

Chapter

8

Meat

Lean Beef Stir-Fry with Broccoli and Peppers

Yield: 4 servings | **Prep time:** 20 minutes | **Cook time:** 10 minutes

- 1 pound lean beef sirloin, thinly sliced
- 4 cups broccoli florets
- 1 red bell pepper, thinly sliced
- 1 yellow bell pepper, thinly sliced
- 2 tablespoons low-sodium soy sauce
- 1 tablespoon olive oil
- 2 cloves garlic, minced
- 1 teaspoon fresh ginger, minced
- 1/4 cup low-sodium beef broth
- Salt and pepper to taste

Nutritional Information:

Approximately 250 calories,   *30g protein,*
12g carbohydrates,   *9g fat,*
60mg cholesterol,   *4g fiber,*
600mg potassium,   *420mg sodium.*

1. In a bowl, mix the low-sodium soy sauce, garlic, and ginger. Add the sliced beef and let it marinate for at least 15 minutes.
2. Heat the olive oil in a large skillet over medium-high heat. Add the marinated beef and stir-fry for about 3 minutes or until cooked to your liking. Remove beef from the skillet and set aside.
3. In the same skillet, add the broccoli and bell peppers. Stir-fry for about 4-5 minutes, or until the vegetables are tender but still crisp.
4. Return the beef to the skillet and add the beef broth. Stir well to combine and let the mixture simmer for 2 minutes.

Lean Beef Stir-Fry with Broccoli and Peppers is a nutritious and heart-healthy meal that combines lean protein with a variety of colorful vegetables. Lean beef sirloin is an excellent source of protein and essential nutrients, while broccoli and bell peppers add fiber, vitamins, and antioxidants to the dish. Using low-sodium soy sauce and broth helps keep the sodium content in check, supporting cardiovascular health. This quick and flavorful stir-fry is perfect for a balanced diet, providing a delicious way to enjoy nutrient-dense ingredients without compromising on taste.

Slow-Cooked Turkey Chili

Yield: 6 servings | **Prep time:** 15 minutes | **Cook time:** 240 minutes

- **1.5 pounds lean ground turkey**
- **1 large onion, diced**
- **3 cloves garlic, minced**
- **1 (15-ounce) can low-sodium black beans, drained and rinsed**
- **1 (15-ounce) can low-sodium kidney beans, drained and rinsed**
- **1 (15-ounce) can low-sodium diced tomatoes, with juice**
- **1 (6-ounce) can tomato paste**
- **1 cup low-sodium chicken or vegetable broth**
- **2 tablespoons chili powder**
- **1 teaspoon cumin**
- **1 teaspoon paprika**
- **Salt and pepper to taste**
- **Optional toppings: diced avocado, chopped cilantro**

1. In a large skillet over medium heat, cook the ground turkey, breaking it up into smaller pieces, until no longer pink. Drain excess fat and transfer to the slow cooker.
2. In the same skillet, sauté the onion and garlic until translucent. Add to the slow cooker.
3. Add the drained beans, diced tomatoes with juice, tomato paste, broth, and spices to the slow cooker. Stir to combine all the ingredients.
4. Cover and cook on low for 4 hours, stirring occasionally. Adjust salt and pepper to taste before serving.

Nutritional Information:

Approximately 320 calories,	*28g protein,*
32g carbohydrates,	*7g fat,*
60mg cholesterol,	*10g fiber,*
600mg potassium,	*420mg sodium.*

Slow-Cooked Turkey Chili is a hearty, nutritious dish perfect for heart-healthy diets. Lean ground turkey serves as a low-fat protein source, while a mix of black and kidney beans adds fiber and essential nutrients. Using low-sodium beans and broth helps manage sodium intake, crucial for heart health. The combination of tomatoes, onions, garlic, and spices like chili powder, cumin, and paprika enriches the chili with antioxidants and anti-inflammatory properties. This dish is not only delicious but also supports cardiovascular wellness, making it a great option for a balanced diet. Serve with optional avocado and cilantro for added flavor and nutrition.

Rosemary-Garlic Grilled Chicken Breast

Yield: 4 servings | **Prep time:** 15 minutes | **Cook time:** 12 minutes

- **4 boneless, skinless chicken breasts (about 6 oz each)**
- **3 cloves garlic, minced**
- **2 tablespoons olive oil**
- **2 tablespoons fresh rosemary, finely chopped**
- **Juice of 1 lemon**
- **Salt and pepper to taste**

Nutritional Information:

Approximately 250 calories,	*30g protein,*
3g carbohydrates,	*13g fat,*
85mg cholesterol,	*0g fiber,*
400mg potassium,	*200mg sodium.*

1. In a bowl, mix together the minced garlic, olive oil, rosemary, and lemon juice. Season with salt and pepper.
2. Place the chicken breasts in a resealable plastic bag or shallow dish. Pour the rosemary-garlic marinade over the chicken, making sure each piece is well-coated. Seal the bag or cover the dish and marinate in the refrigerator for at least 1 hour.
3. Preheat the grill to medium-high heat.
4. Remove the chicken from the marinade and grill for about 6 minutes per side, or until the internal temperature reaches 165°F (75°C).
5. Let the chicken rest for a few minutes before serving.

Rosemary-Garlic Grilled Chicken Breast is a flavorful and heart-healthy dish, perfect for those looking to maintain a balanced diet. Lean chicken breasts provide high-quality protein with minimal fat, supporting muscle maintenance and overall health. The marinade, made with garlic, olive oil, rosemary, and lemon juice, not only enhances the flavor but also offers numerous health benefits. Garlic and rosemary are known for their anti-inflammatory and antioxidant properties, while olive oil and lemon juice contribute to cardiovascular health. This simple yet delicious recipe is a great addition to any heart-healthy diet plan.

Apple-Glazed Pork Loin

Yield: 4 servings | **Prep time:** 20 minutes | **Cook time:** 60 minutes

- **1 pork loin (about 1.5 lbs)**
- **2 tablespoons olive oil**
- **Salt and pepper to taste**
- **1 cup unsweetened applesauce**
- **1 tablespoon apple cider vinegar**
- **2 teaspoons Dijon mustard**
- **1 teaspoon fresh thyme, minced**
- **1 teaspoon fresh rosemary, minced**
- **2 cloves garlic, minced**

Nutritional Information:

Approximately 380 calories,	*35g protein,*
20g carbohydrates,	*16g fat,*
95mg cholesterol,	*2g fiber,*
700mg potassium,	*250mg sodium.*

1. Preheat the oven to 350°F (175°C). Rub the pork loin with olive oil, salt, and pepper. Place it in a baking dish.
2. In a small bowl, mix together the applesauce, apple cider vinegar, Dijon mustard, thyme, rosemary, and garlic.
3. Pour the apple glaze mixture over the pork loin, ensuring it's evenly coated.
4. Cover the baking dish with aluminum foil and bake for 50 minutes. Remove the foil and continue to bake for another 10 minutes or until the internal temperature of the pork reaches 145°F (63°C).
5. Let the pork loin rest for 5 minutes before slicing. Serve warm.

Apple-Glazed Pork Loin offers a delightful blend of savory and sweet flavors, making it an ideal dish for heart-healthy eating. This recipe features lean pork loin, a great source of protein, paired with a delicious apple glaze made from unsweetened applesauce, apple cider vinegar, and herbs. The combination of thyme and rosemary adds a fragrant touch, while the Dijon mustard provides a tangy kick. By using olive oil and minimizing added sugars and sodium, this dish supports cardiovascular health. Enjoy a nutritious, flavorful meal that's perfect for any heart-conscious diet.

Balsamic Glazed Pork Tenderloin

Yield: 4 servings | **Prep time:** 15 minutes | **Cook time:** 25 minutes

- **1 pork tenderloin (about 1.5 pounds)**
- **1/4 cup balsamic vinegar**
- **2 tablespoons olive oil**
- **2 tablespoons honey**
- **1 tablespoon minced garlic**
- **1 teaspoon dried thyme**
- **Salt and pepper to taste**

Nutritional Information:

Approximately 260 calories,	*32g protein,*
13g carbohydrates,	*8g fat,*
80mg cholesterol,	*0g fiber,*
550mg potassium,	*250mg sodium.*

1. Preheat the oven to 400°F (200°C). In a bowl, mix balsamic vinegar, olive oil, honey, garlic, thyme, salt, and pepper to make the glaze.
2. Place the pork tenderloin in a baking dish and pour half of the glaze over it, making sure to coat it evenly. Reserve the remaining glaze for later.
3. Roast the pork in the preheated oven for 20 minutes, occasionally basting with the pan juices.
4. During the last 5 minutes of cooking, pour the remaining glaze over the pork. Finish roasting until the internal temperature reaches at least 145°F (63°C).
5. Remove from oven, let rest for a few minutes, then slice and serve.

Balsamic Glazed Pork Tenderloin is a delightful and heart-healthy dish that combines lean protein with a tangy, slightly sweet glaze. Pork tenderloin is a lean cut of meat, making it a great choice for a heart-healthy diet. The balsamic vinegar and honey glaze adds rich flavor without excessive calories or fat. This dish is also seasoned with garlic and thyme, which not only enhance the taste but also offer additional health benefits. This recipe is simple to prepare and perfect for a nutritious and satisfying meal that supports cardiovascular health

Spiced Lamb Kebabs with Cucumber Yogurt Sauce

Yield: 4 servings | **Prep time:** 30 minutes (including marination) | **Cook time:** 10 minutes

For the Kebabs:
- **1 pound lean lamb, cut into 1-inch cubes**
- **1 tablespoon olive oil**
- **1 teaspoon ground cumin**
- **1 teaspoon ground coriander**
- **1/2 teaspoon ground cinnamon**
- **Salt and pepper to taste**
- **8 wooden or metal skewers**

For the Cucumber Yogurt Sauce:
- **1 cup low-fat Greek yogurt**
- **1 small cucumber, finely diced**
- **1 clove garlic, minced**
- **1 tablespoon fresh lemon juice**
- **Salt and pepper to taste**

1. In a mixing bowl, combine the lamb cubes, olive oil, cumin, coriander, cinnamon, salt, and pepper. Toss well to coat the meat evenly. Cover and marinate in the refrigerator for at least 20 minutes.
2. While the meat is marinating, prepare the Cucumber Yogurt Sauce. Mix together the Greek yogurt, diced cucumber, minced garlic, lemon juice, salt, and pepper. Set aside.
3. Preheat the grill or grill pan over medium-high heat. Thread the marinated lamb cubes onto the skewers.
4. Grill the lamb kebabs for about 4-5 minutes per side, or until cooked to your desired level of doneness.
5. Serve the lamb kebabs with a generous dollop of Cucumber Yogurt Sauce.

Nutritional Information:
Approximately 300 calories, 28g protein, 8g carbohydrates, 16g fat, 70mg cholesterol, 1g fiber, 400mg potassium, 250mg sodium.

Spiced Lamb Kebabs with Cucumber Yogurt Sauce offer a delightful blend of flavors that are both heart-healthy and satisfying. Lean lamb provides a rich source of protein and essential nutrients, while the use of olive oil and aromatic spices like cumin, coriander, and cinnamon enhances the taste without adding unhealthy fats. The accompanying Cucumber Yogurt Sauce made with low-fat Greek yogurt and fresh cucumber adds a refreshing touch, promoting good digestion and providing probiotics for gut health. This dish is a balanced, flavorful option perfect for those following a heart-healthy diet.

Grilled Lemon-Herb Chicken Thighs

Yield: 4 servings | **Prep time:** 15 minutes | **Cook time:** 20 minutes

- **4 boneless, skinless chicken thighs (about 1.5 pounds)**
- **2 lemons, zested and juiced**
- **3 tablespoons olive oil**
- **3 cloves garlic, minced**
- **2 tablespoons fresh thyme leaves (or 1 tablespoon dried)**
- **Salt and pepper to taste**
- **Optional garnish: lemon slices and additional thyme sprigs**

Nutritional Information:
Approximately 320 calories, 28g protein, 4g carbohydrates, 22g fat, 135mg cholesterol, 1g fiber, 340mg potassium, 220mg sodium.

1. In a mixing bowl, combine lemon zest, lemon juice, olive oil, garlic, thyme, salt, and pepper. Mix well.
2. Place chicken thighs in a large zip-top bag or shallow dish. Pour the lemon-herb mixture over the chicken, making sure each piece is well-coated. Seal the bag or cover the dish and marinate in the refrigerator for at least 1 hour, up to overnight.
3. Preheat grill to medium-high heat. Remove chicken from the marinade and discard the marinade.
4. Grill chicken thighs for 10 minutes per side or until they reach an internal temperature of 165°F (74°C).

Grilled Lemon-Herb Chicken Thighs offer a flavorful and heart-healthy option for your meals. The marinade, made with fresh lemon juice, zest, garlic, and thyme, not only imparts a zesty and aromatic flavor but also provides beneficial antioxidants. Grilling the chicken thighs ensures they are cooked with minimal added fats, keeping the dish lean while maintaining moisture and tenderness. This recipe is perfect for a nutritious dinner, offering high protein and healthy fats, contributing to a balanced diet that supports heart health. Serve with a side of vegetables for a complete meal.

Skinless Turkey Meatballs in Marinara

Yield: 4 servings | **Prep time:** 20 minutes | **Cook time:** 30 minutes

- 1 pound lean ground turkey
- 1/2 cup whole grain breadcrumbs
- 1 large egg, beaten
- 2 tablespoons fresh parsley, chopped
- 1 clove garlic, minced
- 1/4 cup grated Parmesan cheese (optional)
- Salt and pepper to taste
- 2 cups low-sodium marinara sauce
- 1 tablespoon olive oil

Nutritional Information:

Approximately 350 calories, 30g protein, 22g carbohydrates, 14g fat, 90mg cholesterol, 4g fiber, 700mg potassium, 600mg sodium.

1. In a large mixing bowl, combine ground turkey, breadcrumbs, beaten egg, parsley, garlic, Parmesan cheese (if using), salt, and pepper. Mix well.
2. Roll the mixture into 1.5-inch meatballs, placing them on a plate or tray.
3. In a large skillet, heat the olive oil over medium heat. Add the meatballs and brown them on all sides, approximately 6-8 minutes.
4. Once the meatballs are browned, pour the marinara sauce over them. Cover and simmer on low heat for about 20 minutes, or until meatballs are cooked through.

Skinless Turkey Meatballs in Marinara is a nutritious and heart-healthy option for those seeking a delicious yet low-fat meal. Made with lean ground turkey, whole grain breadcrumbs, and fresh herbs, these meatballs offer a high protein content while keeping the fat and cholesterol levels low. The use of low-sodium marinara sauce further reduces sodium intake, beneficial for maintaining healthy blood pressure. This dish is not only flavorful but also easy to prepare, making it an excellent choice for a wholesome, balanced diet that supports heart health.

Citrus-Marinated Pork Chops

Yield: 4 servings | **Prep time:** 10 minutes (plus marinating time) | **Cook time:** 12 minutes

- 4 boneless pork chops (about 4 oz each)
- 1 orange, juiced
- 1 lemon, juiced
- 1 lime, juiced
- 2 cloves garlic, minced
- 1 tablespoon olive oil
- Salt and pepper to taste
- 2 tablespoons fresh cilantro, chopped (optional for garnish)

Nutritional Information:

Approximately 260 calories, 25g protein, 5g carbohydrates, 15g fat, 0g fiber, 65mg cholesterol, 100mg sodium, 400mg potassium.

1. In a bowl, combine the orange juice, lemon juice, lime juice, minced garlic, and olive oil. Mix well. Place pork chops in a resealable plastic bag and pour the marinade over them. Seal the bag and marinate for at least 1 hour in the refrigerator.
2. Preheat grill to medium-high heat. Remove pork chops from the marinade and discard the marinade. Season the chops with salt and pepper.
3. Place the pork chops on the grill and cook for about 5-6 minutes per side, or until the internal temperature reaches 145°F (63°C).
4. Remove the pork chops from the grill and let them rest for a few minutes before serving. Garnish with fresh cilantro if desired.

Citrus-Marinated Pork Chops are a flavorful and heart-healthy option for your diet. The tangy marinade, made from fresh orange, lemon, and lime juices, not only infuses the pork chops with a refreshing taste but also adds a boost of vitamin C and antioxidants. Using lean boneless pork chops keeps the dish lower in fat, while the olive oil adds healthy monounsaturated fats beneficial for heart health. This recipe is quick to prepare and perfect for grilling, making it an ideal choice for a nutritious and delicious meal that supports cardiovascular wellness.

Sous-Vide Pork Loin with Cherry Sauce

Yield: 4 servings | **Prep time:** 20 minutes | **Cook time:** 2 hours 30 minutes

- 1.5 lbs pork loin
- 1 tablespoon olive oil
- Salt and pepper to taste
- 1 cup pitted cherries (fresh or frozen)
- 1/4 cup water
- 1 tablespoon balsamic vinegar
- 1 teaspoon fresh rosemary, finely chopped
- 1/4 teaspoon ground cinnamon
- Optional: Fresh rosemary for garnish

Nutritional Information:

Approximately 310 calories, 35g protein, 12g carbohydrates, 12g fat, 90mg cholesterol, 2g fiber, 540mg potassium, 300mg sodium.

1. Preheat the sous-vide machine to 140°F (60°C). Season the pork loin with salt and pepper. Place the pork loin in a vacuum-sealed bag with olive oil and seal it tightly. Sous-vide for 2 hours.
2. In a small saucepan, combine cherries, water, balsamic vinegar, fresh rosemary, and cinnamon. Simmer over low heat for 15-20 minutes, stirring occasionally, until the sauce thickens. Set aside.
3. After the pork loin has finished sous-viding, preheat a skillet on medium-high heat. Remove the pork loin from the bag and sear it on all sides for 2-3 minutes to give it a golden brown finish.
4. Slice the pork loin and serve it with the cherry sauce. Optionally, garnish with a sprig of fresh rosemary.

Sous-Vide Pork Loin with Cherry Sauce offers a balanced and nutritious option for those focusing on heart health. This recipe features tender pork loin cooked sous-vide to retain its natural juices and tenderness, minimizing added fats. The cherry sauce, infused with balsamic vinegar and fresh herbs, provides antioxidants and flavor without excessive sodium. High in protein and potassium, this dish supports heart health while being low in calories and moderate in fat. Enjoy a flavorful meal that nourishes and satisfies, perfect for maintaining a health

Veal Scallopini with Lemon and Capers

Yield: 4 servings | **Prep time:** 15 minutes | **Cook time:** 15 minutes

- 4 veal cutlets (about 4 ounces each), pounded thin
- 2 tablespoons olive oil
- Salt and pepper to taste
- 1/2 cup low-sodium chicken broth
- Juice of 1 lemon
- 2 tablespoons capers, drained and rinsed
- 1 clove garlic, minced
- 1 tablespoon chopped fresh parsley for garnish
- Lemon wedges for serving

Nutritional Information:

Approximately 230 calories, 25g protein, 3g carbohydrates, 12g fat, 80mg cholesterol, 0g fiber, 370mg potassium, 220mg sodium.

1. Heat the olive oil in a large skillet over medium-high heat. Season the veal cutlets with salt and pepper on both sides.
2. Add the veal cutlets to the skillet and cook for 2-3 minutes per side, or until lightly browned. Remove the veal from the skillet and set aside.
3. In the same skillet, add the garlic and sauté for about 30 seconds. Add the chicken broth, lemon juice, and capers. Bring the mixture to a simmer, scraping up any browned bits from the bottom of the skillet.
4. Return the veal to the skillet and simmer in the sauce for another 2-3 minutes, or until the veal is cooked through.
5. Garnish with fresh parsley and serve with lemon wedges on the side.

Veal Scallopini with Lemon and Capers is a delightful and heart-healthy dish that combines tender veal cutlets with a tangy lemon-caper sauce. Veal is a lean source of protein, essential for muscle maintenance and repair, while olive oil provides healthy monounsaturated fats that are beneficial for heart health. The lemon juice adds a fresh, zesty flavor and is a good source of vitamin C, which supports cardiovascular health. Capers and fresh parsley not only enhance the taste but also add antioxidants and anti-inflammatory properties, making this dish a nutritious and delicious choice for a heart-healthy diet.

Baked Chicken with Quinoa and Asparagus

Yield: 4 servings | **Prep time:** 15 minutes | **Cook time:** 30 minutes

- **4 boneless, skinless chicken breasts (about 1.5 lbs)**
- **1 cup uncooked quinoa**
- **2 cups low-sodium chicken broth**
- **1 bunch of asparagus, trimmed and cut into 2-inch pieces**
- **2 tablespoons olive oil**
- **1 lemon, zested and juiced**
- **2 cloves garlic, minced**
- **Salt and pepper to taste**
- **Fresh parsley for garnish (optional)**

Nutritional Information:

Approximately 400 calories,	*40g protein,*
35g carbohydrates,	*10g fat,*
80mg cholesterol,	*5g fiber,*
600mg potassium,	*200mg sodium.*

1. Preheat your oven to 400°F (200°C). In a baking dish, place the chicken breasts and season them with half of the olive oil, lemon zest, lemon juice, minced garlic, salt, and pepper.
2. In a separate dish, mix the quinoa and low-sodium chicken broth. Place the asparagus on top and drizzle with the remaining olive oil. Season with salt and pepper.
3. Cover both dishes with aluminum foil and place them in the preheated oven. Bake the chicken for 25-30 minutes and the quinoa and asparagus for about 20 minutes, or until the quinoa is cooked and the asparagus is tender.
4. Once cooked, plate the chicken alongside a helping of quinoa and asparagus. Garnish with fresh parsley if desired.

Baked Chicken with Quinoa and Asparagus is a wholesome and balanced meal, perfect for a heart-healthy diet. This dish features lean, boneless chicken breasts that provide high-quality protein while being low in saturated fats. Quinoa, a nutrient-dense grain, is rich in fiber and essential amino acids, supporting heart health and digestion. Asparagus adds vitamins and minerals, including folate and antioxidants, which promote cardiovascular wellness. The simple seasoning of lemon, garlic, and olive oil enhances the flavor without adding excessive calories or sodium, making this recipe both delicious and nutritious.

Lemon-Dill Roasted Chicken

Yield: 4 servings | **Prep time:** 15 minutes | **Cook time:** 45 minutes

- **4 boneless, skinless chicken breasts (about 1.5 lbs)**
- **2 tablespoons olive oil**
- **1 large lemon, zested and juiced**
- **2 tablespoons fresh dill, chopped**
- **4 cloves garlic, minced**
- **Salt and pepper to taste**
- **1 pound asparagus, trimmed**
- **1 medium onion, thinly sliced**

Nutritional Information:

Approximately 280 calories,	*35g protein,*
10g carbohydrates,	*12g fat,*
80mg cholesterol,	*3g fiber,*
550mg potassium,	*200mg sodium.*

1. Preheat the oven to 400°F (200°C). In a small bowl, mix together olive oil, lemon zest, lemon juice, dill, garlic, salt, and pepper.
2. Place the chicken breasts in a large baking dish. Drizzle half of the lemon-dill mixture over the chicken, making sure to coat each piece evenly.
3. Arrange the asparagus and sliced onions around the chicken in the baking dish. Drizzle the remaining lemon-dill mixture over the vegetables.
4. Cover the baking dish with aluminum foil and bake for 25 minutes. Remove the foil and bake for an additional 20 minutes, or until the chicken reaches an internal temperature of 165°F (74°C).

Lemon-Dill Roasted Chicken is a delightful, heart-healthy dish that combines the bright flavors of lemon and fresh dill with tender chicken breasts. The addition of asparagus and onions enhances the nutritional profile, providing essential vitamins, minerals, and fiber. This recipe uses olive oil, a source of healthy fats, which supports cardiovascular health. By baking the chicken and vegetables together, the dish ensures a balanced meal that's low in calories but high in protein and nutrients, making it perfect for those following a heart-conscious diet. Enjoy this zesty, nutritious meal that promotes overall well-being.

Jerk-Spiced Turkey Breast

Yield: 4 servings | **Prep time:** 10 minutes | **Cook time:** 35 minutes

- **1 turkey breast (about 1.5 pounds), skinless and boneless**
- **1 tablespoon olive oil**
- **1 tablespoon jerk seasoning (low-sodium preferred)**
- **Juice of 1 lime**
- **2 cloves garlic, minced**
- **1 teaspoon fresh ginger, grated**
- **Salt and pepper to taste**
- **Fresh cilantro leaves, for garnish**

Nutritional Information:

Approximately 220 calories, *42g protein,*
3g carbohydrates, *5g fat,*
90mg cholesterol, *1g fiber,*
420mg potassium, *210mg sodium.*

1. Preheat the oven to 375°F (190°C). Line a baking sheet with parchment paper.
2. In a small bowl, mix together the olive oil, jerk seasoning, lime juice, garlic, and ginger.
3. Rub the seasoning mixture all over the turkey breast, making sure to coat evenly. Season with a pinch of salt and pepper.
4. Place the seasoned turkey breast on the prepared baking sheet. Bake for 30-35 minutes or until the internal temperature reaches 165°F (74°C).
5. Remove from the oven, let it rest for a few minutes, then slice and garnish with fresh cilantro leaves before serving.

Jerk-Spiced Turkey Breast is a flavorful and nutritious option for a heart-healthy diet. Turkey breast is a lean source of high-quality protein, which is essential for muscle maintenance and overall health. The jerk seasoning adds a spicy kick without the need for excessive salt, making it a lower-sodium choice that supports cardiovascular health. Fresh lime juice, garlic, and ginger not only enhance the flavor but also provide antioxidants and anti-inflammatory benefits. This dish is not only delicious but also supports heart health by providing essential nutrients with minimal saturated fat.

Tandoori Chicken with Cilantro-Mint Chutney

Yield: 4 servings | **Prep time:** 20 minutes (plus 2 hours for marination) | **Cook time:** 20 minutes

For the Tandoori Chicken:
- **4 boneless, skinless chicken breasts**
- **1 cup Greek yogurt (low-fat)**
- **2 cloves garlic, minced**
- **1-inch ginger, minced**
- **1 tablespoon lemon juice**
- **1 teaspoon turmeric powder**
- **1 teaspoon ground cumin**
- **1 teaspoon ground coriander**
- **1 teaspoon paprika**
- **Salt to taste**

For the Cilantro-Mint Chutney:
- **1 cup fresh cilantro leaves**
- **1/2 cup fresh mint leaves**
- **1 green chili (optional)**
- **1 tablespoon lemon juice**
- **Salt to taste**

1. In a mixing bowl, combine Greek yogurt, garlic, ginger, lemon juice, turmeric, cumin, coriander, paprika, and salt. Add the chicken breasts and mix until well coated. Cover and marinate for at least 2 hours or overnight for best results.

2. Preheat the grill to medium-high heat. Remove chicken from the marinade and discard any excess marinade. Grill the chicken for about 7-10 minutes on each side, or until the internal temperature reaches 165°F (75°C).
3. While the chicken is grilling, prepare the cilantro-mint chutney. In a blender, add cilantro, mint, green chili (if using), lemon juice, and salt. Blend until smooth.
4. Serve the grilled tandoori chicken hot, accompanied by the cilantro-mint chutney.

Nutritional Information:
Approximately 280 calories,

35g protein,

10g carbohydrates,

9g fat,

2g fiber,

85mg cholesterol,

280mg sodium,

650mg potassium.

Tandoori Chicken with Cilantro-Mint Chutney is a flavorful and heart-healthy dish perfect for those looking to add some spice to their diet. Marinated in a blend of low-fat Greek yogurt, garlic, ginger, and aromatic spices like turmeric, cumin, and coriander, the chicken is grilled to perfection, offering a lean source of protein. The refreshing cilantro-mint chutney adds a vibrant, zesty complement, enhancing the dish with fresh herbs and lemon juice. This combination not only tantalizes your taste buds but also supports cardiovascular health with its low-fat, nutrient-rich ingredients. Enjoy a delicious meal that's both satisfying and good for your heart.

Sesame-Crusted Chicken with Steamed Vegetables

Yield: 4 servings | **Prep time:** 15 minutes | **Cook time:** 20 minutes

- **4 boneless, skinless chicken breasts (about 6 oz each)**
- **1/2 cup sesame seeds**
- **1 tablespoon olive oil**
- **Salt and pepper to taste**
- **1/2 teaspoon garlic powder**
- **2 cups broccoli florets**
- **1 cup sliced carrots**
- **1 cup snap peas**
- **1 tablespoon low-sodium soy sauce**

1. Preheat oven to 375°F (190°C). Line a baking sheet with parchment paper or lightly grease it.
2. In a shallow bowl, mix sesame seeds, garlic powder, salt, and pepper. Dip each chicken breast in the mixture, pressing gently to adhere the sesame seeds to all sides.
3. In a skillet, heat olive oil over medium heat. Sear each chicken breast for about 2 minutes per side or until the sesame seeds are golden.
4. Transfer the seared chicken breasts to the prepared baking sheet. Bake for 15-18 minutes or until the chicken is cooked through.
5. While the chicken is baking, steam broccoli, carrots, and snap peas until tender-crisp, about 5 minutes. Drizzle with low-sodium soy sauce before serving.

Nutritional Information:

Approximately 360 calories,	*40g protein,*
12g carbohydrates,	*16g fat,*
95mg cholesterol,	*5g fiber,*
650mg potassium,	*280mg sodium.*

Sesame-Crusted Chicken with Steamed Vegetables is a perfect dish for heart health, combining lean protein with nutrient-dense veggies. The sesame seeds provide healthy fats and antioxidants, while the chicken breasts are a great source of lean protein, supporting muscle maintenance and overall health. Steaming the broccoli, carrots, and snap peas ensures they retain their vitamins and minerals, such as fiber, vitamin C, and potassium, which are vital for heart health and blood pressure regulation. This low-sodium, low-carb meal is delicious and beneficial for maintaining a healthy cardiovascular system.

Herbed Roast Beef with Root Vegetables

Yield: 4 servings | **Prep time:** 20 minutes | **Cook time:** 60 minutes

- **1.5 pounds lean beef roast (such as sirloin tip roast)**
- **2 tablespoons olive oil**
- **1 tablespoon chopped fresh rosemary**
- **1 tablespoon chopped fresh thyme**
- **2 cloves garlic, minced**
- **Salt and pepper to taste**
- **4 medium carrots, peeled and cut into chunks**
- **4 medium parsnips, peeled and cut into chunks**
- **1 large onion, quartered**
- **2 tablespoons balsamic vinegar**

Nutritional Information:

Approximately 400 calories,	*40g protein,*
30g carbohydrates,	*14g fat,*
90mg cholesterol,	*6g fiber,*
800mg potassium,	*220mg sodium.*

1. Preheat the oven to 400°F (200°C). In a small bowl, combine olive oil, rosemary, thyme, garlic, salt, and pepper to create the herb mixture.
2. Rub the herb mixture all over the beef roast, making sure it's evenly coated.
3. In a roasting pan, place the coated beef roast in the center and surround it with the cut carrots, parsnips, and onion. Drizzle the vegetables with balsamic vinegar.
4. Cover the roasting pan with aluminum foil and roast for 45 minutes. Remove the foil and continue roasting for an additional 15 minutes or until the beef reaches your desired level of doneness.
5. Remove from the oven and let the beef rest for about 10 minutes before slicing. Serve the sliced beef alongside the roasted vegetables.

Herbed Roast Beef with Root Vegetables is a hearty and nutritious dish perfect for a heart-healthy diet. Lean beef roast, such as sirloin tip, is seasoned with fresh rosemary, thyme, garlic, and olive oil, providing a flavorful and low-fat protein source. Roasting the beef with a medley of carrots, parsnips, and onion, drizzled with balsamic vinegar, adds a rich, caramelized flavor while packing in essential vitamins, minerals, and fiber. This balanced meal supports cardiovascular health by offering a mix of lean protein, healthy fats, and nutrient-dense vegetables, making it an excellent choice for those focused on heart wellness.

Thai-Style Beef Salad

Yield: 4 servings | **Prep time:** 25 minutes | **Cook time:** 10 minutes

For the Salad:
- **1 lb lean sirloin beef steak**
- **4 cups mixed salad greens (e.g., romaine, arugula, spinach)**
- **1 medium cucumber, thinly sliced**
- **1 medium carrot, julienned**
- **1 red bell pepper, thinly sliced**
- **1/2 cup fresh cilantro leaves**
- **1/4 cup fresh mint leaves**

For the Dressing:
- **3 tablespoons fresh lime juice**
- **2 tablespoons low-sodium soy sauce**
- **1 tablespoon fish sauce**
- **1 teaspoon grated ginger**
- **1 garlic clove, minced**
- **1 teaspoon honey or agave syrup**
- **1/4 teaspoon crushed red pepper flakes (optional)**

1. Preheat your grill or grill pan to medium-high heat. Grill the sirloin steak for 5 minutes per side or until it reaches your desired level of doneness. Let it rest for 5 minutes before slicing thinly against the grain.
2. While the beef is resting, prepare the salad ingredients. In a large bowl, combine the mixed greens, cucumber, carrot, bell pepper, cilantro, and mint.
3. To make the dressing, whisk together the lime juice, low-sodium soy sauce, fish sauce, grated ginger, minced garlic, honey, and crushed red pepper flakes (if using).
4. Toss the salad with half of the dressing. Divide the salad among four plates. Top with sliced beef and drizzle the remaining dressing over the top.

Nutritional Information:

Approximately 270 calories,	*30g protein,*
18g carbohydrates,	*8g fat,*
55mg cholesterol,	*4g fiber,*
750mg potassium,	*320mg sodium.*

Thai-Style Beef Salad is a vibrant and refreshing dish that perfectly balances flavors and textures, making it an ideal choice for a heart-healthy diet. Lean sirloin steak, grilled to perfection, provides a rich source of protein while mixed greens, cucumber, carrot, and red bell pepper offer a variety of vitamins and antioxidants. Fresh herbs like cilantro and mint add an aromatic touch. The tangy dressing, made with lime juice, low-sodium soy sauce, and a hint of honey, enhances the overall flavor without adding excessive sodium or sugar. This nutritious salad is light, flavorful, and great for maintaining cardiovascular health.

Buffalo Chicken Stuffed Sweet Potatoes

Yield: 4 servings | **Prep time:** 15 minutes | **Cook time:** 45 minutes

- **4 medium sweet potatoes**
- **2 chicken breasts (about 8 oz each)**
- **1/2 cup low-sodium chicken broth**
- **1/4 cup hot sauce (e.g., Frank's RedHot)**
- **1 teaspoon olive oil**
- **1 small onion, diced**
- **2 cloves garlic, minced**
- **Salt and pepper to taste**
- **2 green onions, sliced for garnish**
- **1/4 cup low-fat Greek yogurt (optional, for topping)**

Nutritional Information:

Approximately 320 calories,	*28g protein,*
40g carbohydrates,	*4g fat,*
60mg cholesterol,	*6g fiber,*
800mg potassium,	*600mg sodium.*

1. Preheat oven to 400°F (200°C). Pierce each sweet potato a few times with a fork and place on a baking sheet. Bake for 40-45 minutes or until tender.
2. While the sweet potatoes are baking, cook chicken breasts in chicken broth in a covered pan over medium heat. Cook for 15-20 minutes or until fully cooked. Shred the chicken using two forks.
3. In a skillet, heat olive oil over medium heat. Add diced onion and garlic, cooking until translucent. Add the shredded chicken, hot sauce, salt, and pepper, stirring to combine.
4. Cut each baked sweet potato lengthwise to create a pocket, being careful not to cut all the way through. Stuff with the buffalo chicken mixture.
5. Garnish with green onions and a dollop of low-fat Greek yogurt if desired.

Buffalo Chicken Stuffed Sweet Potatoes offer a flavorful and nutritious twist on a classic dish, making it an excellent choice for a heart-healthy diet. Sweet potatoes are rich in fiber, vitamins A and C, and potassium, which contribute to maintaining a healthy heart and regulating blood pressure. The lean chicken breast provides a high-protein, low-fat filling, while the buffalo sauce adds a spicy kick without excess calories. Topping it with low-fat Greek yogurt enhances the dish with probiotics and additional protein, making this a well-rounded, delicious meal that supports cardiovascular health.

Balsamic Chicken and Mushroom Skillet

Yield: 4 servings | **Prep time:** 15 minutes | **Cook time:** 20 minutes

- **4 boneless, skinless chicken breasts (about 1.5 lbs)**
- **1 tablespoon olive oil**
- **1 lb button mushrooms, sliced**
- **1 medium onion, diced**
- **3 cloves garlic, minced**
- **1/2 cup low-sodium chicken broth**
- **1/4 cup balsamic vinegar**
- **1 tablespoon fresh thyme leaves (or 1 teaspoon dried thyme)**
- **Salt and pepper to taste**
- **Optional: 1 tablespoon chopped fresh parsley for garnish**

Nutritional Information:

Approximately 310 calories,	*40g protein,*
12g carbohydrates,	*10g fat,*
95mg cholesterol,	*2g fiber,*
650mg potassium,	*220mg sodium.*

1. Heat the olive oil in a large skillet over medium-high heat. Season the chicken breasts with salt and pepper. Add them to the skillet and cook for about 5-6 minutes per side, or until they are cooked through. Remove the chicken and set aside.
2. In the same skillet, add the mushrooms, onion, and garlic. Sauté for 5 minutes or until the mushrooms are browned and the onions are translucent.
3. Add the balsamic vinegar, low-sodium chicken broth, and thyme to the skillet. Bring to a simmer and let it cook for 3-4 minutes, allowing the flavors to meld and the sauce to slightly thicken.
4. Return the cooked chicken to the skillet and simmer in the sauce for another 2-3 minutes, making sure the chicken is well-coated.
5. Optional: Garnish with fresh parsley before serving.

Balsamic Chicken and Mushroom Skillet is a heart-healthy dish that aligns perfectly with the "Heart Health Diet". This recipe features lean chicken breasts cooked in olive oil, accompanied by nutrient-rich mushrooms and onions. The addition of balsamic vinegar not only enhances the flavor but also provides antioxidants that support cardiovascular health. With low-sodium chicken broth and minimal fat, it's a balanced meal that's low in calories and high in protein, essential for maintaining a healthy heart. Enjoy this savory skillet as a delicious way to care for your heart without sacrificing flavor.

Barbecue Chicken with Pineapple Coleslaw

Yield: 4 servings | **Prep time:** 20 minutes | **Cook time:** 20 minutes

For the chicken:
- **4 boneless, skinless chicken breasts (around 4-5 oz each)**
- **1 cup low-sodium barbecue sauce**
- **1 tablespoon olive oil**

For the Pineapple Coleslaw:
- **3 cups shredded cabbage**
- **1 cup diced pineapple**
- **1/4 cup shredded carrots**
- **1/4 cup low-fat Greek yogurt**
- **1 tablespoon apple cider vinegar**
- **1 teaspoon honey**
- **Salt and pepper to taste**

1. Preheat the grill to medium-high heat. While the grill is heating, brush the chicken breasts with olive oil and season with salt and pepper. Once the grill is ready, grill the chicken breasts for about 7-8 minutes per side, or until the internal temperature reaches 165°F.

2. While the chicken is grilling, prepare the pineapple coleslaw. In a large bowl, combine the shredded cabbage, diced pineapple, and shredded carrots.
3. In a separate bowl, whisk together the low-fat Greek yogurt, apple cider vinegar, honey, salt, and pepper. Pour the dressing over the cabbage mixture and toss to combine.
4. Once the chicken is done, generously brush each piece with low-sodium barbecue sauce and grill for an additional 1-2 minutes per side to caramelize the sauce.
5. Serve each grilled chicken breast with a generous helping of pineapple coleslaw.

Nutritional Information:

Approximately 320 calories,	*30g protein,*
35g carbohydrates,	*6g fat,*
75mg cholesterol,	*4g fiber,*
520mg potassium,	*400mg sodium.*

Barbecue Chicken with Pineapple Coleslaw is a flavorful and nutritious dish ideal for those looking to maintain a balanced diet. Grilled boneless, skinless chicken breasts are brushed with low-sodium barbecue sauce, offering a lean protein source that supports muscle health. The pineapple coleslaw, featuring shredded cabbage, diced pineapple, and carrots, provides a crunchy texture along with vitamins and fiber. Tossed in a light dressing of low-fat Greek yogurt, apple cider vinegar, and honey, the coleslaw adds a refreshing contrast to the savory chicken. Enjoy this satisfying meal that's low in calories and sodium, making it a perfect choice for a healthy lifestyle.

Skillet Chicken Fajitas with Whole Wheat Tortillas

Yield: 4 servings | **Prep time:** 15 minutes | **Cook time:** 15 minutes

- **1 pound boneless, skinless chicken breasts, sliced into thin strips**
- **1 tablespoon olive oil**
- **1 large red bell pepper, sliced**
- **1 large green bell pepper, sliced**
- **1 medium-sized onion, sliced**
- **2 cloves garlic, minced**
- **1 teaspoon ground cumin**
- **1 teaspoon paprika**
- **Salt and pepper to taste**
- **Juice of 1 lime**
- **4 whole-wheat tortillas**
- **Fresh cilantro leaves, for garnish**

1. Heat olive oil in a large skillet over medium heat. Add the sliced bell peppers, onion, and garlic. Cook until the vegetables are softened, about 5-7 minutes.
2. Add the sliced chicken breast to the skillet. Season with ground cumin, paprika, salt, and pepper. Cook until the chicken is no longer pink, about 5-8 minutes.
3. Stir in the lime juice and cook for an additional 2 minutes.
4. Warm the whole-wheat tortillas in a separate pan or in the microwave for about 30 seconds.
5. Serve the chicken and vegetable mixture in the warm whole-wheat tortillas, garnished with fresh cilantro leaves.

Nutritional Information:

Approximately 340 calories,	*28g protein,*
30g carbohydrates,	*12g fat,*
65mg cholesterol,	*4g fiber,*
500mg potassium,	*450mg sodium.*

Skillet Chicken Fajitas with Whole Wheat Tortillas are a heart-healthy meal packed with lean protein and fiber-rich vegetables. Using skinless chicken breast reduces saturated fat intake, while bell peppers and onions provide essential vitamins and antioxidants. Whole wheat tortillas add extra fiber, supporting healthy digestion and heart function. Seasoned with cumin and paprika, and finished with fresh lime juice, these fajitas offer a flavorful, balanced meal that's low in sodium and high in nutrients. Perfect for maintaining a heart-healthy diet without sacrificing taste.

Asian-Style Lettuce Wraps with Ground Chicken

Yield: 4 servings | **Prep time:** 20 minutes | **Cook time:** 10 minutes

- 1 pound lean ground chicken
- 1 tablespoon olive oil
- 1 small onion, finely diced
- 2 cloves garlic, minced
- 1 red bell pepper, diced
- 1 cup shredded carrots
- 1/4 cup low-sodium soy sauce
- 2 teaspoons rice vinegar
- 1 teaspoon ground ginger
- 1 teaspoon chili flakes (optional for heat)
- 8 large lettuce leaves (Bibb or Iceberg)
- Optional toppings: chopped scallions, fresh cilantro, lime wedges

1. Heat the olive oil in a large skillet over medium heat. Add the onions and garlic and sauté until translucent.
2. Add the ground chicken to the skillet, breaking it apart with a spatula. Cook until the chicken is no longer pink.
3. Stir in the diced red bell pepper and shredded carrots. Cook for another 2-3 minutes.
4. Add the soy sauce, rice vinegar, ground ginger, and chili flakes (if using). Stir well to combine and cook for an additional 2 minutes.
5. Spoon the chicken mixture into the lettuce leaves and garnish with optional toppings if desired.

Nutritional Information:
Approximately 280 calories,
26g protein,
14g carbohydrates,
10g fat,
3g fiber,
70mg cholesterol,
400mg sodium,
500mg potassium,

Asian-Style Lettuce Wraps with Ground Chicken offer a light and flavorful meal perfect for a heart-healthy diet. Lean ground chicken provides high-quality protein while keeping fat content low. Using lettuce leaves instead of traditional wraps reduces carbohydrates and adds a refreshing crunch. The inclusion of vegetables like red bell pepper and carrots boosts fiber and essential vitamins, supporting cardiovascular health. Low-sodium soy sauce helps manage sodium intake, crucial for maintaining healthy blood pressure levels. This dish combines nutritious ingredients with aromatic spices, creating a satisfying and heart-friendly meal option.

Always remember to add only a minimal amount of salt to the recipe !
Or replace salt with spices on page 10

HEART HEALTHY

— ★★★★★ —

DIET

Chapter

9

Side Dishes

Steamed Green Beans with Almond Slivers

Yield: 4 servings | **Prep time:** 10 minutes | **Cook time:** 10 minutes

- **1 pound fresh green beans, trimmed**
- **1 tablespoon olive oil**
- **2 tablespoons almond slivers**
- **Salt and pepper to taste**
- **1 teaspoon lemon zest (optional)**
- **1 tablespoon lemon juice (optional)**

Nutritional Information:
Approximately 80 calories,

3g protein,

9g carbohydrates,

4g fat,

4g fiber,

0mg cholesterol,

80mg sodium,

240mg potassium.

1. Bring a pot of water to a boil and prepare a steamer basket. Place the green beans in the steamer basket and steam for 5-7 minutes, or until they reach your desired level of tenderness.
2. In a skillet, heat olive oil over medium heat. Add the almond slivers and sauté until they turn golden brown, about 2-3 minutes.
3. Toss the steamed green beans and almond slivers together in a serving bowl.
4. Optionally, add lemon zest and lemon juice for extra flavor. Season with salt and pepper to taste before serving.

Steamed Green Beans with Almond Slivers is a simple and nutritious side dish perfect for a heart-healthy diet. Fresh green beans are steamed to retain their vibrant color and nutrients, while almond slivers sautéed in olive oil add a delightful crunch and healthy fats. For an extra burst of flavor, lemon zest and juice can be added, providing a refreshing citrus note. This dish is low in calories and high in fiber, making it an excellent choice for maintaining cardiovascular health while enjoying a delicious and wholesome meal.

Quinoa-Stuffed Bell Peppers

Yield: 4 servings | **Prep time:** 20 minutes | **Cook time:** 40 minutes

- **4 large bell peppers, halved and seeds removed**
- **1 cup quinoa, rinsed and drained**
- **2 cups low-sodium vegetable broth**
- **1 tablespoon olive oil**
- **1 small onion, diced**
- **2 cloves garlic, minced**
- **1 can (14.5 oz) diced tomatoes, drained**
- **1 teaspoon ground cumin**
- **Salt and pepper to taste**
- **1 cup cooked black beans (canned or freshly cooked)**
- **1 cup chopped fresh spinach**
- **1/4 cup chopped fresh cilantro (optional for garnish)**

Nutritional Information:

Approximately 290 calories,	*11g protein,*
50g carbohydrates,	*6g fat,*
0mg cholesterol,	*9g fiber,*
700mg potassium,	*280mg sodium.*

1. Preheat your oven to 375°F (190°C). Place the halved bell peppers cut-side up in a baking dish.
2. In a medium saucepan, combine quinoa and vegetable broth. Bring to a boil, reduce heat, cover, and simmer for 15 minutes or until the quinoa is cooked. Fluff with a fork and set aside.
3. While the quinoa is cooking, heat olive oil in a skillet over medium heat. Add onions and garlic, and sauté until translucent. Stir in the diced tomatoes and cumin. Season with salt and pepper.
4. Combine the cooked quinoa, black beans, and spinach with the onion-tomato mixture. Stir well to mix.
5. Spoon the quinoa mixture into each bell pepper half. Cover the baking dish with aluminum foil and bake for 25 minutes or until the peppers are tender.

Quinoa-Stuffed Bell Peppers are a hearty and nutritious option perfect for a heart-healthy diet. Packed with protein-rich quinoa and black beans, this dish offers a balanced blend of fiber, vitamins, and minerals. Fresh spinach and diced tomatoes add antioxidants and essential nutrients, while the use of low-sodium vegetable broth and minimal added salt helps keep sodium levels in check. These stuffed peppers are low in fat and cholesterol-free, making them an ideal choice for maintaining cardiovascular health. Enjoy this colorful and delicious meal that's both satisfying and good for your heart.

Garlic and Rosemary Sweet Potato Wedges

Yield: 4 servings | **Prep time:** 15 minutes | **Cook time:** 30 minutes

- **2 large sweet potatoes, washed and cut into wedges**
- **2 tablespoons olive oil**
- **3 cloves garlic, minced**
- **1 tablespoon fresh rosemary, finely chopped**
- **Salt and pepper to taste**

Nutritional Information:

Approximately 200 calories,	*2g protein,*
28g carbohydrates,	*9g fat,*
0mg cholesterol,	*4g fiber,*
450mg potassium,	*90mg sodium.*

1. Preheat your oven to 400°F (200°C). Line a baking sheet with parchment paper.
2. In a large mixing bowl, combine sweet potato wedges, olive oil, minced garlic, and rosemary. Toss well to coat all the wedges.
3. Spread the sweet potato wedges evenly on the prepared baking sheet, avoiding overlap. Season with salt and pepper to taste.
4. Bake for 30 minutes, flipping the wedges halfway through, until they are golden brown and crisp on the edges.

Garlic and Rosemary Sweet Potato Wedges make a delicious and heart-healthy side dish. Sweet potatoes are rich in vitamins, fiber, and antioxidants, supporting overall cardiovascular health. Tossed with olive oil, minced garlic, and fresh rosemary, these wedges offer a flavorful and aromatic twist. Baking instead of frying keeps them lower in fat while still achieving a crispy texture. Low in sodium and cholesterol-free, this dish is perfect for those looking to enjoy a nutritious and satisfying meal that benefits heart health.

Oven-Roasted Garlic Asparagus

Yield: 4 servings | Prep time: 10 minutes | Cook time: 15 minutes

- 1 pound fresh asparagus spears, trimmed
- 2 tablespoons olive oil
- 4 cloves garlic, minced
- Salt to taste (optional)
- Freshly ground black pepper to taste
- Zest of 1 lemon (for garnish, optional)

Nutritional Information:
Approximately 85 calories,
2g protein,
6g carbohydrates,
7g fat,
2g fiber,
0mg cholesterol,
230mg potassium,
200mg sodium.

1. Preheat your oven to 400°F (200°C). Line a baking sheet with parchment paper for easy cleanup.
2. Place the asparagus on the prepared baking sheet, ensuring they are spread out in a single layer. Drizzle the olive oil over the asparagus and sprinkle the minced garlic evenly on top. If using salt, lightly sprinkle it along with the freshly ground black pepper over the asparagus.
3. Use your hands or a pair of tongs to toss and coat the asparagus evenly with the olive oil, garlic, salt, and pepper.
4. Roast in the preheated oven for about 12-15 minutes or until the asparagus are tender but still crisp. Cooking time may vary depending on the thickness of the asparagus spears.
5. If desired, finish by adding lemon zest over the roasted asparagus for an added burst of flavor before serving.

Oven-Roasted Garlic Asparagus is a simple yet delicious dish that perfectly complements a heart-healthy diet. Fresh asparagus spears are coated with olive oil and minced garlic, then roasted to tender perfection, enhancing their natural flavors. This dish is rich in fiber, vitamins, and antioxidants, while olive oil adds heart-healthy fats. A sprinkle of lemon zest can be added for a fresh burst of flavor. Low in calories and carbohydrates, this asparagus recipe makes a nutritious and tasty side dish for any meal, promoting overall cardiovascular health.

Lemon and Herb Couscous

Yield: 4 servings | Prep time: 10 minutes | Cook time: 10 minutes

- 1 cup whole-grain couscous
- 1 1/4 cups low-sodium vegetable broth
- 1 tablespoon olive oil
- Zest of 1 lemon
- Juice of 1/2 lemon
- 1/4 cup chopped fresh parsley
- 1/4 cup chopped fresh mint
- Salt and pepper to taste

Nutritional Information:
Approximately 210 calories,   *6g protein,*
40g carbohydrates,   *3g fat,*
0mg cholesterol,   *4g fiber,*
180mg potassium,   *150mg sodium.*

1. In a medium saucepan, bring the low-sodium vegetable broth to a boil.
2. Stir in the couscous, cover, and remove from heat. Let it sit for 5 minutes, or until all the liquid is absorbed.
3. Fluff the couscous with a fork and transfer it to a large mixing bowl.
4. Add the olive oil, lemon zest, lemon juice, chopped parsley, and chopped mint. Mix well to combine. Season with salt and pepper to taste.
5. Serve warm or at room temperature, as a side or part of a main dish.

Lemon and Herb Couscous is a light and flavorful side dish perfect for a heart-healthy diet. Made with whole-grain couscous, this dish provides essential fiber and nutrients that support cardiovascular health. The addition of fresh parsley and mint adds a burst of antioxidants, while lemon zest and juice give a refreshing, tangy flavor. Using low-sodium vegetable broth keeps the sodium content low, and olive oil adds healthy fats. Enjoy this versatile dish warm or at room temperature, enhancing any meal with its vibrant taste and heart-healthy benefits.

Mediterranean Chickpea Salad

Yield: 4 servings | **Prep time:** 15 minutes | **Cook time:** 0 minutes

- 1 can (15 ounces) chickpeas, drained and rinsed
- 1 cup cherry tomatoes, halved
- 1 cucumber, diced
- 1/2 red onion, finely chopped
- 1/4 cup kalamata olives, pitted and sliced
- 1/4 cup feta cheese, crumbled (optional)
- 2 tablespoons olive oil
- Juice of 1 lemon
- 1 teaspoon dried oregano
- Salt and pepper to taste
- 1/4 cup fresh parsley, chopped (for garnish)

Nutritional Information:

Approximately 230 calories,   *8g protein,*

25g carbohydrates,   *12g fat,*

0mg cholesterol,   *7g fiber,*

300mg potassium,   *450mg sodium.*

1. In a large bowl, combine chickpeas, cherry tomatoes, cucumber, red onion, kalamata olives, and feta cheese (if using).
2. In a separate small bowl, whisk together olive oil, lemon juice, and dried oregano. Season with salt and pepper to taste.
3. Pour the dressing over the salad and toss well to combine.
4. Garnish with fresh parsley before serving. The salad can be eaten immediately or refrigerated for up to 2 days for better flavor melding.

Mediterranean Chickpea Salad is a vibrant, heart-healthy dish perfect for any meal. Chickpeas provide a rich source of plant-based protein and fiber, essential for cardiovascular health. Fresh vegetables like cherry tomatoes, cucumber, and red onion add vitamins and antioxidants, while kalamata olives and a drizzle of olive oil contribute healthy fats. The tangy dressing made from lemon juice and oregano enhances the flavors, and optional feta cheese adds a creamy texture. Low in calories and high in nutrients, this salad is a delicious and nutritious option for those looking to support heart health.

Cumin-Spiced Carrot and Parsnip Fries

Yield: 4 servings | **Prep time:** 15 minutes | **Cook time:** 25 minutes

- 3 large carrots, peeled and cut into fries
- 3 large parsnips, peeled and cut into fries
- 2 tablespoons olive oil
- 1 teaspoon ground cumin
- Salt and pepper to taste

Nutritional Information:

Approximately 160 calories,

2g protein,

25g carbohydrates,

7g fat,

6g fiber,

0mg cholesterol,

80mg sodium,

490mg potassium.

1. Preheat your oven to 425°F (220°C). Line a baking sheet with parchment paper.
2. In a large mixing bowl, combine the carrot and parsnip fries with olive oil and ground cumin. Toss well to coat.
3. Spread the carrot and parsnip fries evenly on the prepared baking sheet, avoiding overlap. Season with salt and pepper to taste.
4. Bake for 25 minutes, flipping the fries halfway through, until they are golden brown and crispy at the edges.

Cumin-Spiced Carrot and Parsnip Fries are a delicious and heart-healthy alternative to traditional fries. Carrots and parsnips are rich in vitamins, fiber, and antioxidants, supporting cardiovascular health and overall wellness. Coated in olive oil and seasoned with ground cumin, these fries offer a unique and flavorful twist. Baking them keeps the dish low in fat while achieving a crispy texture. Low in sodium and free from cholesterol, these fries make a nutritious and tasty side dish, perfect for those aiming to maintain a heart-healthy diet.

Balsamic-Glazed Brussels Sprouts

Yield: 4 servings | **Prep time:** 10 minutes | **Cook time:** 25 minutes

- **1 lb Brussels sprouts, trimmed and halved**
- **2 tablespoons olive oil**
- **Salt and pepper to taste**
- **1/4 cup balsamic vinegar**
- **1 tablespoon honey or maple syrup (optional, for added sweetness)**

Nutritional Information:
Approximately 120 calories,

3g protein,

14g carbohydrates,

6g fat,

4g fiber,

0mg cholesterol,

24mg sodium,

440mg potassium.

1. Preheat your oven to 400°F (200°C). Line a baking sheet with parchment paper.
2. In a mixing bowl, toss the Brussels sprouts with olive oil, salt, and pepper. Spread them out evenly on the prepared baking sheet.
3. Roast in the preheated oven for 20 minutes, or until Brussels sprouts are golden and slightly crispy on the edges.
4. While the Brussels sprouts are roasting, prepare the balsamic glaze by reducing the balsamic vinegar in a small saucepan over low heat until it thickens. Optionally, add honey or maple syrup for sweetness.
5. Drizzle the balsamic glaze over the roasted Brussels sprouts before serving.

Balsamic-Glazed Brussels Sprouts are a tasty and heart-healthy addition to any meal. Brussels sprouts are packed with fiber, vitamins, and antioxidants that support cardiovascular health. Roasting them with olive oil enhances their natural flavors and adds healthy fats. The balsamic glaze, optionally sweetened with honey or maple syrup, provides a delicious tangy finish. Low in calories and sodium, and free of cholesterol, this dish offers a nutritious and flavorful way to enjoy more vegetables, making it an excellent choice for a heart-conscious diet.

Zesty Lime and Cilantro Cauliflower Rice

Yield: 4 servings | **Prep time:** 10 minutes | **Cook time:** 10 minutes

- **1 large head of cauliflower, grated (about 4 cups)**
- **1 tablespoon olive oil**
- **1 small onion, finely chopped**
- **2 cloves garlic, minced**
- **Juice of 1 lime**
- **1/2 cup cilantro leaves, chopped**
- **Salt and pepper to taste**

Nutritional Information:
Approximately 80 calories, *3g protein,*

12g carbohydrates, *3g fat,*

0mg cholesterol, *4g fiber,*

350mg potassium, *100mg sodium.*

1. Heat the olive oil in a large skillet over medium heat. Add the chopped onion and minced garlic. Sauté until the onion is translucent, about 3 minutes.
2. Add the grated cauliflower to the skillet. Stir well to combine with the onions and garlic.
3. Cover and cook for about 5-7 minutes, stirring occasionally, until the cauliflower rice is tender but not mushy.
4. Remove from heat and stir in the lime juice and chopped cilantro. Season with salt and pepper to taste.
5. Serve immediately, either as a main or a side dish.

Zesty Lime and Cilantro Cauliflower Rice is a flavorful and heart-healthy dish that's perfect as a main or side. Cauliflower, a low-calorie vegetable rich in fiber and vitamins, is transformed into a rice-like texture and combined with aromatic onions and garlic. The addition of lime juice and fresh cilantro provides a zesty, refreshing flavor, while olive oil adds healthy fats. This dish is low in carbohydrates and sodium, making it an excellent choice for those aiming to maintain a heart-healthy diet without compromising on taste. Enjoy this nutritious, easy-to-make recipe for a delicious and health-conscious meal.

Grilled Corn with Chili-Lime Butter

Yield: 4 servings | **Prep time:** 10 minutes | **Cook time:** 15 minutes

- 4 ears of corn, husked and cleaned
- 1 tablespoon olive oil
- 2 tablespoons unsalted butter, softened
- Zest of 1 lime
- Juice of 1/2 lime
- 1/2 teaspoon chili powder
- Salt to taste
- Fresh cilantro leaves for garnish (optional)

Nutritional Information:

Approximately 180 calories,	3g protein,
27g carbohydrates,	8g fat,
15mg cholesterol,	3g fiber,
250mg potassium,	200mg sodium.

1. Preheat your grill to medium-high heat. Brush each ear of corn lightly with olive oil.
2. In a small bowl, mix the softened butter, lime zest, lime juice, chili powder, and salt. Set aside.
3. Place the corn on the preheated grill. Cook for 12-15 minutes, turning occasionally, until the corn is evenly charred and tender.
4. Remove the corn from the grill and immediately spread the chili-lime butter mixture over each ear.
5. Garnish with cilantro leaves if desired, and serve immediately.

Grilled Corn with Chili-Lime Butter is a flavorful and heart-healthy side dish that's perfect for any barbecue. Fresh ears of corn are brushed with olive oil and grilled to bring out their natural sweetness and achieve a smoky char. The chili-lime butter, made with softened unsalted butter, lime zest, lime juice, and chili powder, adds a zesty and slightly spicy kick. This dish is relatively low in calories and provides fiber, vitamins, and minerals essential for maintaining cardiovascular health. Garnish with fresh cilantro for an added burst of freshness and enjoy this delicious and nutritious summer treat.

Roasted Beets and Arugula Salad

Yield: 4 servings | **Prep time:** 15 minutes | **Cook time:** 45 minutes

- 4 medium-sized beets, peeled and cut into wedges
- 1 tablespoon olive oil
- Salt and pepper to taste
- 4 cups arugula leaves, washed and dried
- 1/4 cup crumbled feta cheese (optional, for a dairy-free option, omit or use dairy-free cheese)
- 1/4 cup walnuts, lightly toasted
- 1 tablespoon balsamic vinegar
- 2 tablespoons extra-virgin olive oil

Nutritional Information:

Approximately 220 calories,	5g protein,
16g carbohydrates,	16g fat,
10mg cholesterol,	4g fiber,
400mg potassium,	180mg sodium.

1. Preheat the oven to 400°F (200°C). Toss the beet wedges with 1 tablespoon of olive oil, salt, and pepper. Place them on a baking sheet lined with parchment paper.
2. Roast the beets in the preheated oven for about 45 minutes, or until they are tender. Remove from oven and let them cool.
3. In a large salad bowl, combine the arugula, cooled roasted beets, feta cheese (if using), and walnuts.
4. In a small bowl, whisk together the balsamic vinegar and 2 tablespoons of extra-virgin olive oil. Drizzle the dressing over the salad and toss to combine.
5. Serve immediately, or refrigerate for later use.

Roasted Beets and Arugula Salad is a vibrant and nutritious dish perfect for a heart-healthy diet. The earthy sweetness of roasted beets pairs beautifully with the peppery arugula, creating a balanced and flavorful salad. Walnuts add a satisfying crunch and healthy fats, while optional feta cheese provides a creamy contrast. A simple balsamic vinaigrette enhances the flavors without adding excessive calories. Rich in fiber, antioxidants, and essential nutrients, this salad supports cardiovascular health and makes a delicious addition to any meal. Enjoy it fresh or refrigerated for later use.

Curried Butternut Squash Soup

Yield: 4 servings | **Prep time:** 15 minutes | **Cook time:** 45 minutes

- **1 medium butternut squash, peeled, seeded, and cubed (about 4 cups)**
- **1 tablespoon olive oil**
- **1 medium onion, chopped**
- **2 cloves garlic, minced**
- **1 tablespoon curry powder**
- **4 cups low-sodium vegetable broth**
- **Salt and pepper to taste**
- **Optional: Fresh cilantro leaves for garnish**

Nutritional Information:

Approximately 150 calories,	*2g protein,*
30g carbohydrates,	*3g fat,*
0mg cholesterol,	*5g fiber,*
700mg potassium,	*150mg sodium.*

1. Heat olive oil in a large pot over medium heat. Add the chopped onion and garlic and sauté until translucent, about 5 minutes.
2. Stir in the curry powder and cook for an additional 1-2 minutes, or until fragrant.
3. Add the cubed butternut squash and vegetable broth to the pot. Bring to a boil, then reduce heat to low, cover, and simmer for about 30-35 minutes, or until the squash is tender.
4. Use an immersion blender or a regular blender to purée the soup until smooth. If using a regular blender, be sure to allow the soup to cool slightly and blend in batches.
5. Season with salt and pepper to taste, and garnish with fresh cilantro leaves if desired.

Curried Butternut Squash Soup is a warm and comforting dish ideal for a heart-healthy diet. Butternut squash is rich in vitamins, fiber, and antioxidants, supporting overall cardiovascular health. The addition of curry powder adds a flavorful spice blend that enhances the natural sweetness of the squash. Using low-sodium vegetable broth helps keep the sodium content in check. This soup is low in calories and fat while being high in essential nutrients like potassium. Enjoy this creamy and nutritious soup, garnished with fresh cilantro for a burst of freshness, perfect for a healthy and satisfying meal.

Stir-Fried Snow Peas and Red Peppers

Yield: 4 servings | **Prep time:** 10 minutes | **Cook time:** 8 minutes

- **2 cups snow peas, trimmed**
- **1 large red bell pepper, sliced into thin strips**
- **1 tablespoon olive oil**
- **2 cloves garlic, minced**
- **1 tablespoon low-sodium soy sauce**
- **1 teaspoon sesame seeds (optional)**
- **Salt and pepper to taste**

Nutritional Information:

Approximately 80 calories,	2g protein,
10g carbohydrates,	3g fat,
0mg cholesterol,	3g fiber,
300mg potassium,	200mg sodium.

1. Heat olive oil in a large skillet or wok over medium-high heat.
2. Add the minced garlic and sauté for about 30 seconds, or until fragrant.
3. Add the snow peas and red bell pepper strips to the skillet. Stir-fry for about 5-7 minutes, or until the vegetables are tender-crisp.
4. Stir in the low-sodium soy sauce and cook for another 1 minute.
5. Season with salt and pepper to taste, and sprinkle with sesame seeds if using. Serve immediately.

Stir-Fried Snow Peas and Red Peppers is a quick and nutritious dish perfect for a heart-healthy diet. This vibrant stir-fry features snow peas and red bell peppers, both rich in vitamins, antioxidants, and fiber, supporting cardiovascular health. Sautéed in olive oil with garlic for added flavor, the vegetables remain tender-crisp, preserving their nutrients. A touch of low-sodium soy sauce enhances the taste without adding excessive sodium. Optional sesame seeds provide a hint of nuttiness. Low in calories and cholesterol-free, this dish makes a delicious and healthy side or light main course.

Sautéed Spinach with Garlic and Lemon

Yield: 4 servings | **Prep time:** 5 minutes | **Cook time:** 5 minutes

- **10 ounces fresh spinach leaves, washed and drained**
- **2 tablespoons olive oil**
- **3 cloves garlic, minced**
- **Zest of 1 lemon**
- **Juice of half a lemon**
- **Salt and pepper to taste**

Nutritional Information:

Approximately 90 calories, *3g protein,*
4g carbohydrates, *7g fat,*
0mg cholesterol, *2g fiber,*
500mg potassium, *200mg sodium*

1. In a large skillet, heat olive oil over medium heat.
2. Add minced garlic and sauté for about 1 minute, or until fragrant but not browned.
3. Add the spinach leaves to the skillet. Use tongs to turn the leaves so that they wilt evenly. This should take about 3 minutes.
4. Add lemon zest and lemon juice, and toss to combine.
5. Season with salt and pepper to taste. Serve immediately.

Sautéed Spinach with Garlic and Lemon is a simple yet flavorful dish ideal for a heart-healthy diet. Fresh spinach is rich in iron, vitamins, and antioxidants, supporting overall cardiovascular health. Sautéed in olive oil, the spinach absorbs the aromatic flavors of garlic, while lemon zest and juice add a refreshing citrus note. This dish is low in calories and carbohydrates, with healthy fats from olive oil, making it a nutritious and quick side dish that complements any meal. Enjoy this vibrant and nutrient-packed recipe for a delicious boost to your heart health.

Parmesan Zucchini Noodles

Yield: 4 servings | **Prep time:** 10 minutes | **Cook time:** 5 minutes

- **4 medium zucchinis, spiralized into noodles**
- **2 tablespoons olive oil**
- **2 cloves garlic, minced**
- **1/4 cup grated Parmesan cheese**
- **Salt and pepper to taste**
- **Fresh basil leaves for garnish (optional)**

Nutritional Information:

Approximately 130 calories,
6g protein,
8g carbohydrates,
10g fat,
2g fiber,
5mg cholesterol,
180mg sodium,
500mg potassium.

1. Spiralize the zucchinis into noodles and set them aside.
2. In a large skillet, heat olive oil over medium heat. Add minced garlic and sauté for about 1 minute, or until fragrant.
3. Add the zucchini noodles to the skillet and sauté for 2-3 minutes, just until tender.
4. Turn off the heat and sprinkle the grated Parmesan over the zucchini noodles. Toss well to combine.
5. Season with salt and pepper to taste. Garnish with fresh basil leaves if desired. Serve immediately.

Parmesan Zucchini Noodles are a light and healthy alternative to traditional pasta, perfect for a heart-healthy diet. Zucchini, spiralized into noodles, provides a low-carb, nutrient-rich base high in vitamins and antioxidants. Sautéed briefly in olive oil with garlic, these noodles are tender yet firm. The addition of grated Parmesan adds a rich, savory flavor without excessive calories. This dish is low in sodium and cholesterol-free, making it a delicious and nutritious choice for those looking to maintain cardiovascular health. Enjoy this quick and easy meal, garnished with fresh basil for an extra burst of flavor.

Smoky Paprika Roasted Potatoes

Yield: 4 servings | **Prep time:** 15 minutes | **Cook time:** 35 minutes

- **4 medium-sized russet potatoes, washed and cut into wedges**
- **2 tablespoons olive oil**
- **1 tablespoon smoked paprika**
- **1 teaspoon garlic powder**
- **Salt and pepper to taste**
- **Fresh parsley for garnish (optional)**

Nutritional Information:
Approximately 220 calories,
4g protein,
40g carbohydrates,
6g fat, 3g fiber,
0mg cholesterol,
10mg sodium,
800mg potassium.

1. Preheat the oven to 400°F (200°C). Line a baking sheet with parchment paper.
2. In a large bowl, combine the potato wedges, olive oil, smoked paprika, and garlic powder. Toss until the potatoes are well-coated.
3. Spread the coated potato wedges evenly on the prepared baking sheet, making sure they are not overcrowded.
4. Roast in the preheated oven for 30-35 minutes, turning halfway through, until the potatoes are golden and crisp.
5. Remove from the oven, season with salt and pepper to taste, and garnish with fresh parsley if desired.

Smoky Paprika Roasted Potatoes are a flavorful and heart-healthy side dish perfect for any meal. Russet potatoes are rich in potassium and fiber, supporting cardiovascular health. Coated in olive oil, smoked paprika, and garlic powder, these potatoes are roasted to golden perfection, offering a delicious smoky flavor without excessive fat. Low in cholesterol and high in essential nutrients, this dish makes a nutritious and satisfying addition to your diet. Garnish with fresh parsley for a touch of freshness and enjoy these crispy, savory potato wedges.

Maple and Mustard Glazed Carrots

Yield: 4 servings | **Prep time:** 10 minutes | **Cook time:** 25 minutes

- **1 pound baby carrots, washed and peeled**
- **2 tablespoons pure maple syrup**
- **1 tablespoon Dijon mustard**
- **1 tablespoon olive oil**
- **Salt and pepper to taste**
- **Fresh parsley for garnish (optional)**

Nutritional Information:
Approximately 120 calories,   *1g protein,*
24g carbohydrates,   *3g fat,*
0mg cholesterol,   *3g fiber,*
350mg potassium,   *160mg sodium,*

1. Preheat your oven to 400°F (200°C). Line a baking sheet with parchment paper.
2. In a bowl, mix together the maple syrup, Dijon mustard, and olive oil.
3. Add the baby carrots to the bowl and toss them until they are well-coated with the maple-mustard mixture.
4. Spread the carrots evenly on the prepared baking sheet. Roast for 20-25 minutes or until tender, stirring once halfway through the cooking time.
5. Remove from oven, season with salt and pepper to taste, and garnish with fresh parsley if desired.

Maple and Mustard Glazed Carrots are a delightful and heart-healthy side dish. Baby carrots, naturally rich in vitamins and fiber, are coated in a flavorful blend of pure maple syrup, Dijon mustard, and olive oil. Roasting enhances their natural sweetness and creates a tender texture. This dish is low in calories and cholesterol-free, making it an excellent choice for those aiming to maintain a heart-healthy diet. The combination of maple and mustard provides a unique sweet and tangy flavor, while a sprinkle of fresh parsley adds a touch of freshness. Enjoy these glazed carrots as a nutritious and delicious complement to any meal.

HEART HEALTHY

— ★★★★★ —

DIET

Chapter

10

Soups

Roasted Tomato and Basil Soup

Yield: 4 servings | **Prep time:** 15 minutes | **Cook time:** 45 minutes

- 8 large tomatoes, quartered
- 1 large onion, chopped
- 4 cloves garlic, minced
- 1/4 cup fresh basil leaves, finely chopped
- 2 tablespoons olive oil
- 4 cups low-sodium vegetable broth
- Salt and pepper to taste
- Optional: 1 teaspoon balsamic vinegar for added flavor

Nutritional Information:

Approximately 150 calories,	*4g protein,*
20g carbohydrates,	*7g fat,*
0mg cholesterol,	*4g fiber,*
750mg potassium,	*180mg sodium.*

1. Preheat the oven to 400°F (200°C). Place the quartered tomatoes on a baking sheet, drizzle with 1 tablespoon of olive oil, and season with salt and pepper. Roast for 25-30 minutes.
2. In a large pot, heat the remaining 1 tablespoon of olive oil over medium heat. Add the chopped onion and garlic and sauté until translucent.
3. Add the roasted tomatoes to the pot along with the low-sodium vegetable broth. Bring to a simmer and cook for 10-15 minutes.
4. Turn off the heat and add the chopped basil leaves. Use an immersion blender to purée the soup until smooth, or transfer to a blender to purée and then return to the pot.
5. Optional: Add 1 teaspoon of balsamic vinegar for additional flavor, if desired. Adjust salt and pepper to taste. Serve hot.

Roasted Tomato and Basil Soup is a heart-healthy, flavorful option perfect for any meal. Roasting the tomatoes intensifies their natural sweetness, while fresh basil adds a fragrant, herbaceous note. This soup is rich in antioxidants, vitamins, and fiber, supporting cardiovascular health. Using low-sodium vegetable broth keeps the sodium content low, and a touch of olive oil adds healthy fats. Optionally, a splash of balsamic vinegar can enhance the depth of flavor. With minimal calories and a robust nutritional profile, this smooth and satisfying soup is a delicious way to enjoy a nutrient-packed meal.

Lentil and Spinach Soup

Yield: 4 servings | **Prep time:** 10 minutes | **Cook time:** 40 minutes

- **1 cup green lentils, rinsed and drained**
- **1 tablespoon olive oil**
- **1 medium onion, chopped**
- **3 cloves garlic, minced**
- **4 cups low-sodium vegetable broth**
- **1 teaspoon ground cumin**
- **1/2 teaspoon ground coriander**
- **Salt and pepper to taste**
- **4 cups baby spinach leaves**
- **Optional: lemon wedges for serving**

Nutritional Information:

Approximately 220 calories,	*12g protein,*
35g carbohydrates,	*4g fat,*
0mg cholesterol,	*15g fiber,*
600mg potassium,	*120mg sodium.*

1. Heat olive oil in a large pot over medium heat. Add the chopped onion and minced garlic. Sauté until the onion is translucent, about 5 minutes.
2. Add the lentils, ground cumin, ground coriander, and vegetable broth to the pot. Bring to a boil, then reduce the heat to low and simmer for 30-35 minutes or until the lentils are tender.
3. Use an immersion blender or potato masher to partially puree the soup, leaving some lentils whole for texture.
4. Add the baby spinach leaves and cook just until wilted, about 2-3 minutes. Season with salt and pepper to taste.
5. Optional: Serve hot, with a wedge of lemon on the side for added flavor.

Lentil and Spinach Soup is a hearty and nutritious choice perfect for a heart-healthy diet. Packed with green lentils, this soup offers a rich source of protein and fiber, which supports cardiovascular health and helps maintain healthy cholesterol levels. Baby spinach adds a dose of vitamins and antioxidants, while ground cumin and coriander provide a warm, earthy flavor. Using low-sodium vegetable broth keeps the sodium content low, and a touch of olive oil adds healthy fats. Enjoy this flavorful and satisfying soup, optionally enhanced with a squeeze of lemon for a refreshing twist.

Mediterranean Chickpea and Lemon Soup

Yield: 4 servings | **Prep time:** 15 minutes | **Cook time:** 25 minutes

- **4 cups low-sodium vegetable broth**
- **2 cans (15 oz each) chickpeas, drained and rinsed**
- **1 large lemon, zested and juiced**
- **1 medium onion, diced**
- **3 cloves garlic, minced**
- **2 tablespoons olive oil**
- **1 teaspoon ground cumin**
- **1 teaspoon ground coriander**
- **Salt and pepper to taste**
- **Optional: Fresh parsley or mint for garnish**

Nutritional Information:

Approximately 260 calories,	*11g protein,*
35g carbohydrates,	*8g fat,*
0mg cholesterol,	*9g fiber,*
400mg potassium,	*300mg sodium.*

1. In a large pot, heat olive oil over medium heat. Add the diced onion and garlic, and sauté until translucent, about 5 minutes.
2. Add the ground cumin and coriander to the pot, stirring to coat the onions and garlic.
3. Stir in the chickpeas, and then add the low-sodium vegetable broth. Bring the mixture to a boil.
4. Lower the heat to a simmer and add the lemon juice and lemon zest. Cook for another 15-20 minutes.
5. Season with salt and pepper to taste. Optional: Garnish with fresh parsley or mint before serving.

Mediterranean Chickpea and Lemon Soup is a vibrant and heart-healthy dish perfect for any occasion. Packed with protein-rich chickpeas, this soup offers a satisfying and nutritious meal. The bright flavors of lemon zest and juice add a refreshing tang, while ground cumin and coriander provide warm, aromatic notes. Using low-sodium vegetable broth ensures a lower sodium content, supporting cardiovascular health. Olive oil adds healthy fats, and a garnish of fresh parsley or mint enhances the flavor and presentation. Enjoy this flavorful soup that's both delicious and beneficial for maintaining a heart-healthy diet.

Beet and Ginger Detox Soup

Yield: 4 servings | **Prep time:** 20 minutes | **Cook time:** 40 minutes

- **4 medium-sized beets, peeled and chopped**
- **1 medium carrot, peeled and chopped**
- **1 small onion, diced**
- **2 cloves garlic, minced**
- **1-inch piece of fresh ginger, peeled and grated**
- **4 cups low-sodium vegetable broth**
- **1 tablespoon olive oil**
- **Juice of half a lemon**
- **Salt and pepper to taste**
- **Optional: Fresh parsley for garnish**

Nutritional Information:

Approximately 120 calories,	*3g protein,*
22g carbohydrates,	*3g fat,*
0mg cholesterol,	*5g fiber,*
450mg potassium,	*200mg sodium.*

1. Heat olive oil in a large pot over medium heat. Add onion, garlic, and ginger, sautéing until the onion becomes translucent, about 5 minutes.
2. Add the chopped beets and carrots to the pot, stirring to combine with the onion mixture.
3. Pour in the low-sodium vegetable broth and bring the mixture to a boil. Reduce the heat to a simmer and cook until the beets and carrots are tender, about 30-35 minutes.
4. Use an immersion blender or a regular blender to purée the soup until smooth. Return the soup to the pot if you used a regular blender.
5. Add the lemon juice, and season with salt and pepper to taste. Optional: Garnish with fresh parsley before serving.

Beet and Ginger Detox Soup is a nourishing and heart-healthy option perfect for a cleanse. Beets are rich in antioxidants, vitamins, and minerals that support liver function and cardiovascular health. The addition of fresh ginger adds a warm, spicy note and aids digestion. Carrots and garlic contribute additional nutrients and flavor, while low-sodium vegetable broth keeps the soup light and low in sodium. A squeeze of lemon juice enhances the taste with a refreshing citrus note. Enjoy this vibrant, smooth soup, optionally garnished with fresh parsley, for a detoxifying and health-boosting meal.

Sweet Corn and Bell Pepper Chowder

Yield: 4 servings | **Prep time:** 15 minutes | **Cook time:** 25 minutes

- **4 cups low-sodium vegetable broth**
- **3 cups fresh sweet corn kernels (about 4 ears)**
- **1 red bell pepper, diced**
- **1 yellow bell pepper, diced**
- **1 small onion, diced**
- **2 cloves garlic, minced**
- **1 medium potato, peeled and diced**
- **2 tablespoons olive oil**
- **1 teaspoon paprika**
- **Salt and pepper to taste**
- **Optional: Fresh parsley for garnish**

Nutritional Information:

Approximately 220 calories,	*6g protein,*
40g carbohydrates,	*5g fat,*
0mg cholesterol,	*6g fiber,*
600mg potassium,	*150mg sodium.*

1. In a large pot, heat olive oil over medium heat. Add the onion and garlic, and sauté until translucent, about 3-5 minutes.
2. Add the bell peppers and potato to the pot and sauté for another 5 minutes.
3. Stir in the corn kernels and paprika, then add the low-sodium vegetable broth. Bring to a boil.
4. Reduce heat and simmer for 15-20 minutes, or until the vegetables are tender.
5. Use a ladle to remove about 2 cups of the chowder and blend until smooth. Return the blended portion back to the pot, stir well, and season with salt and pepper to taste. Optional: Garnish with fresh parsley before serving.

Sweet Corn and Bell Pepper Chowder is a delightful, heart-healthy dish bursting with vibrant flavors and colors. Fresh sweet corn and diced bell peppers provide a rich source of vitamins, fiber, and antioxidants, while potatoes add a creamy texture and additional nutrients. The use of low-sodium vegetable broth ensures the chowder remains low in sodium, supporting cardiovascular health. Olive oil adds healthy fats, and a touch of paprika gives the chowder a warm, smoky flavor. This nutritious and satisfying soup, optionally garnished with fresh parsley, makes for a comforting and wholesome meal.

Vegetable Minestrone with Whole-Grain Pasta

Yield: 4 servings | **Prep time:** 20 minutes | **Cook time:** 30 minutes

- **4 cups low-sodium vegetable broth**
- **1 can (14.5 oz) diced tomatoes, no salt added**
- **1 cup whole-grain elbow pasta**
- **1 medium zucchini, diced**
- **1 medium carrot, diced**
- **1 medium onion, chopped**
- **2 cloves garlic, minced**
- **1 cup green beans, chopped**
- **1 can (15 oz) cannellini beans, drained and rinsed**
- **1 teaspoon dried basil**
- **1 teaspoon dried oregano**
- **1 tablespoon olive oil**
- **Salt and pepper to taste**
- **Optional: Fresh basil leaves for garnish**

1. In a large pot, heat olive oil over medium heat. Add onion and garlic and sauté until translucent, about 3-4 minutes.
2. Add carrots, zucchini, and green beans to the pot. Sauté for another 5 minutes.
3. Pour in the low-sodium vegetable broth and diced tomatoes (with their juice). Add dried basil and dried oregano. Bring to a boil, then reduce heat to low and simmer for 20 minutes.
4. Stir in the whole-grain elbow pasta and cannellini beans. Cook for another 10 minutes or until the pasta is al dente.
5. Season with salt and pepper to taste. Optional: Garnish with fresh basil leaves before serving.

Nutritional Information:

Approximately 280 calories,	*10g protein,*
45g carbohydrates,	*5g fat,*
0mg cholesterol,	*9g fiber,*
400mg potassium,	*150mg sodium.*

Vegetable Minestrone with Whole-Grain Pasta is a hearty and nutritious soup perfect for a heart-healthy diet. Packed with a variety of vegetables like zucchini, carrots, and green beans, this minestrone provides essential vitamins, minerals, and fiber. Whole-grain elbow pasta and cannellini beans add complex carbohydrates and protein, making the soup satisfying and energizing. Using low-sodium vegetable broth and no-salt-added diced tomatoes keeps the sodium content low. Olive oil adds healthy fats, while dried basil and oregano enhance the flavor. Enjoy this delicious, well-balanced soup, optionally garnished with fresh basil leaves, for a wholesome and heart-friendly meal.

Low-Sodium Chicken Noodle Soup

Yield: 4 servings | **Prep time:** 15 minutes | **Cook time:** 25 minutes

- **2 chicken breasts, boneless and skinless (about 1 lb)**
- **6 cups low-sodium chicken broth**
- **2 cups wide egg noodles**
- **1 cup carrots, diced**
- **1 cup celery, diced**
- **1 medium onion, chopped**
- **2 cloves garlic, minced**
- **1 tablespoon olive oil**
- **1/2 teaspoon dried thyme**
- **1/2 teaspoon dried oregano**
- **Salt and pepper to taste**
- **Optional: Chopped fresh parsley for garnish**

1. In a large pot, heat olive oil over medium heat. Add the chopped onion, garlic, carrots, and celery. Sauté for about 5 minutes, or until the vegetables start to soften.

2. Add the chicken breasts, dried thyme, dried oregano, and low-sodium chicken broth to the pot. Bring to a boil, then reduce the heat and simmer for about 20 minutes or until the chicken is cooked through.
3. Remove the chicken breasts from the pot and shred them using two forks. Return the shredded chicken to the pot.
4. Add the wide egg noodles to the pot and cook for 5-7 minutes or until the noodles are tender. Season with salt and pepper to taste.
5. Optional: Garnish with chopped fresh parsley before serving.

Nutritional Information:

Approximately 300 calories,	*30g protein,*
25g carbohydrates,	*7g fat,*
70mg cholesterol,	*2g fiber,*
400mg potassium,	*150mg sodium.*

Low-Sodium Chicken Noodle Soup is a comforting and heart-healthy option perfect for any meal. This classic soup features tender chicken breasts, hearty egg noodles, and a mix of nutritious vegetables like carrots, celery, and onion. Using low-sodium chicken broth keeps the sodium levels in check, while dried thyme and oregano add depth of flavor without the need for extra salt. A touch of olive oil provides healthy fats, and optional fresh parsley adds a burst of freshness. With its balanced mix of protein, carbohydrates, and fiber, this soup is both delicious and nourishing, supporting overall cardiovascular health.

Turkey and Vegetable Barley Soup

Yield: 6 servings | **Prep time:** 20 minutes | **Cook time:** 40 minutes

- **1 lb ground turkey breast**
- **1 cup pearl barley**
- **1 large onion, diced**
- **2 carrots, diced**
- **2 celery stalks, diced**
- **1 zucchini, diced**
- **1 red bell pepper, diced**
- **4 cloves garlic, minced**
- **8 cups low-sodium chicken or vegetable broth**
- **2 tablespoons olive oil**
- **1 teaspoon dried thyme**
- **1 teaspoon dried oregano**
- **Salt and pepper to taste**
- **Optional: Fresh parsley for garnish**

1. In a large pot, heat olive oil over medium heat. Add ground turkey and cook until no longer pink. Break it apart into crumbles as it cooks.
2. Add the diced onion, carrots, celery, and garlic to the pot. Sauté for about 5 minutes, or until the vegetables start to soften.
3. Stir in the barley, zucchini, red bell pepper, thyme, oregano, and low-sodium broth. Bring the mixture to a boil.
4. Reduce the heat to low, cover, and simmer for about 30-35 minutes, or until the barley is tender.
5. Season with salt and pepper to taste. Optionally, garnish with fresh parsley before serving.

Nutritional Information:

Approximately 280 calories,	*28g protein,*
35g carbohydrates,	*5g fat,*
40mg cholesterol,	*8g fiber,*
750mg potassium,	*240mg sodium.*

Turkey and Vegetable Barley Soup is a hearty and nutritious dish perfect for a heart-healthy diet. Ground turkey breast provides lean protein, while a variety of vegetables like carrots, celery, zucchini, and red bell pepper offer essential vitamins and minerals. Pearl barley adds a chewy texture and fiber, aiding digestion and heart health. Using low-sodium broth keeps the sodium content in check, and aromatic herbs like thyme and oregano enhance the flavor. This soup is filling and flavorful, making it an excellent choice for a balanced, heart-conscious meal. Garnish with fresh parsley for an added burst of freshness.

Spiced Pumpkin and Butternut Squash Soup

Yield: 4 servings | **Prep time:** 20 minutes | **Cook time:** 40 minutes

- **2 cups pumpkin puree (canned or fresh)**
- **2 cups butternut squash, peeled and cubed**
- **4 cups low-sodium vegetable broth**
- **1 medium onion, diced**
- **2 cloves garlic, minced**
- **1 teaspoon ground cinnamon**
- **1/2 teaspoon ground nutmeg**
- **1/4 teaspoon ground cloves**
- **1 tablespoon olive oil**
- **Salt and pepper to taste**
- **Optional: Fresh cilantro leaves for garnish**

Nutritional Information:

Approximately 140 calories,	3g protein,
30g carbohydrates,	3g fat,
0mg cholesterol,	6g fiber,
550mg potassium,	80mg sodium.

1. In a large pot, heat olive oil over medium heat. Add onions and garlic, and sauté until translucent, about 5 minutes.
2. Add butternut squash cubes to the pot and sauté for another 5 minutes.
3. Stir in pumpkin puree, ground cinnamon, ground nutmeg, and ground cloves. Add low-sodium vegetable broth. Bring to a boil, then reduce heat and simmer for 30 minutes or until the squash is tender.
4. Use an immersion blender or transfer the soup to a blender and blend until smooth.
5. Season with salt and pepper to taste. Optional: Garnish with fresh cilantro leaves before serving.

Spiced Pumpkin and Butternut Squash Soup is a warm, comforting dish perfect for a heart-healthy diet. This soup combines the rich flavors of pumpkin and butternut squash with aromatic spices like cinnamon, nutmeg, and cloves, creating a deliciously spiced profile. High in fiber and low in calories, this soup supports cardiovascular health while providing essential vitamins and minerals. Using low-sodium vegetable broth helps keep the sodium content in check, and a touch of olive oil adds healthy fats. Enjoy this smooth, flavorful soup, optionally garnished with fresh cilantro, for a nutritious and heartwarming meal.

Curried Cauliflower and Carrot Soup

Yield: 4 servings | **Prep time:** 15 minutes | **Cook time:** 25 minutes

- **1 medium head cauliflower, cut into florets**
- **4 large carrots, peeled and sliced**
- **1 medium onion, diced**
- **3 cloves garlic, minced**
- **4 cups low-sodium vegetable broth**
- **1 can (14 oz) light coconut milk**
- **2 tablespoons olive oil**
- **1 tablespoon curry powder**
- **1 teaspoon ground turmeric**
- **1/2 teaspoon ground cumin**
- **Salt and pepper to taste**
- **Optional: Fresh cilantro for garnish**

1. In a large pot, heat olive oil over medium heat. Add the onion and garlic, sautéing until the onion becomes translucent.
2. Add the carrots and cauliflower to the pot, followed by the curry powder, turmeric, and cumin. Stir to coat the vegetables with the spices.

3. Pour in the low-sodium vegetable broth and bring the mixture to a boil. Reduce heat and let it simmer for about 20 minutes, or until the vegetables are tender.
4. Once the vegetables are cooked, use an immersion blender or stand blender to purée the soup until smooth.
5. Stir in the light coconut milk and season with salt and pepper to taste. Optional: Garnish with fresh cilantro before serving.

Nutritional Information:

Approximately 210 calories,

6g protein,

27g carbohydrates,

10g fat,

8g fiber,

0mg cholesterol,

320mg sodium,

900mg potassium.

Curried Cauliflower and Carrot Soup is a flavorful and heart-healthy dish. This creamy soup combines cauliflower and carrots with aromatic spices like curry powder, turmeric, and cumin, enhancing their natural sweetness and providing anti-inflammatory benefits. The light coconut milk adds a smooth texture while keeping the soup low in cholesterol. Using low-sodium vegetable broth ensures a heart-friendly option. Packed with fiber, vitamins, and minerals, this soup supports overall health. Garnish with fresh cilantro for an extra burst of flavor and enjoy a nutritious meal that's both satisfying and beneficial for your heart.

HEART HEALTHY

— ★★★★★ —

DIET

Chapter

11

Vegetarian Dishes

Broccoli and Cheddar-Stuffed Sweet Potatoes

Yield: 4 servings | **Prep time:** 15 minutes | **Cook time:** 45 minutes

- **4 medium sweet potatoes**
- **2 cups of broccoli florets**
- **1 tablespoon olive oil**
- **1 cup low-fat cheddar cheese, shredded**
- **Salt and pepper to taste**
- **1 teaspoon garlic powder**
- **1/4 teaspoon paprika (optional)**

Nutritional Information:
Approximately 330 calories,
12g protein,
53g carbohydrates,
8g fat,
10g fiber,
20mg cholesterol,
360mg sodium,
800mg potassium.

1. Preheat the oven to 400°F (200°C). Pierce the sweet potatoes with a fork multiple times and place them on a baking sheet lined with parchment paper.
2. Roast the sweet potatoes for 40-45 minutes or until tender when pierced with a fork.
3. While the sweet potatoes are roasting, toss the broccoli florets in olive oil and sprinkle with salt, pepper, and garlic powder. Spread them out on another baking sheet and roast for 15-20 minutes or until tender.
4. Once the sweet potatoes are done, let them cool for a few minutes. Carefully slice each one open lengthwise and fluff the insides with a fork.
5. Stuff each sweet potato with roasted broccoli and top with shredded cheddar cheese. If desired, sprinkle a bit of paprika for color and extra flavor. Serve immediately.

Broccoli and Cheddar-Stuffed Sweet Potatoes is a delicious and heart-healthy meal. Sweet potatoes are roasted to tender perfection, then stuffed with roasted broccoli florets seasoned with garlic powder. Topped with low-fat cheddar cheese, this dish provides a balance of protein, fiber, and essential nutrients. The combination of sweet potatoes and broccoli offers a rich source of vitamins and minerals, supporting overall cardiovascular health. Low in fat and high in potassium, this satisfying and nutritious meal is perfect for a wholesome dinner. Add a sprinkle of paprika for extra flavor and color.

Stuffed Portobello Mushrooms with Quinoa and Spinach

Yield: 4 servings | **Prep time:** 20 minutes | **Cook time:** 30 minutes

- **4 large Portobello mushrooms, stems and gills removed**
- **1 cup cooked quinoa**
- **2 cups fresh spinach, roughly chopped**
- **1 medium onion, finely diced**
- **2 cloves garlic, minced**
- **1 tablespoon olive oil**
- **1/2 cup low-fat feta cheese, crumbled**
- **Salt and pepper to taste**
- **Optional: Fresh herbs (such as parsley or thyme) for garnish**

Nutritional Information:

Approximately 200 calories,	*9g protein,*
25g carbohydrates,	*8g fat,*
10mg cholesterol,	*5g fiber,*
400mg potassium,	*200mg sodium.*

1. Preheat the oven to 375°F (190°C). Line a baking sheet with parchment paper and place the cleaned Portobello mushrooms, cap-side down, on it.
2. In a skillet over medium heat, add olive oil, diced onion, and garlic. Sauté until softened, about 5 minutes.
3. Add the chopped spinach to the skillet and cook until wilted, about 3 minutes. Combine the spinach mixture with cooked quinoa and crumbled feta cheese. Season with salt and pepper to taste.
4. Stuff each Portobello mushroom cap with the quinoa-spinach mixture, pressing down gently to pack the filling.
5. Bake the stuffed mushrooms in the preheated oven for about 20-25 minutes or until the mushrooms are tender and the filling is heated through. Optionally, garnish with fresh herbs before serving.

Stuffed Portobello Mushrooms with Quinoa and Spinach is a nutritious and heart-healthy dish. Large Portobello mushrooms serve as the perfect base, filled with a flavorful mix of quinoa, spinach, onion, and garlic. The addition of low-fat feta cheese adds a savory touch while keeping the dish light. Rich in protein, fiber, and essential nutrients, this meal supports cardiovascular health and overall well-being. Baked to perfection, these stuffed mushrooms are both satisfying and delicious. Optionally, garnish with fresh herbs for an extra burst of flavor and enjoy this wholesome and balanced meal.

Stir-Fried Tofu with Sesame and Broccoli

Yield: 4 servings | **Prep time:** 15 minutes | **Cook time:** 10 minutes

- **1 block (14 ounces) extra-firm tofu, drained and cubed**
- **4 cups broccoli florets**
- **1 tablespoon sesame oil**
- **2 cloves garlic, minced**
- **1/4 cup low-sodium soy sauce**
- **1 tablespoon sesame seeds**
- **1 teaspoon red pepper flakes (optional for heat)**
- **Salt to taste**

Nutritional Information:

Approximately 210 calories,	*18g protein,*
12g carbohydrates,	*10g fat,*
0mg cholesterol,	*4g fiber,*
500mg potassium,	*400mg sodium.*

1. Press the tofu with paper towels to remove excess moisture. Cut into cubes.
2. Heat sesame oil in a large skillet or wok over medium-high heat. Add the minced garlic and sauté for about 1 minute until fragrant.
3. Add the cubed tofu to the skillet and stir-fry for about 5 minutes, or until lightly golden.
4. Add the broccoli florets to the skillet, and continue to stir-fry for another 3-5 minutes or until the broccoli is tender but still crisp.
5. Pour in the low-sodium soy sauce and toss to combine. Sprinkle with sesame seeds, red pepper flakes (if using), and salt to taste. Stir well before serving.

Stir-Fried Tofu with Sesame and Broccoli is a nutritious and heart-healthy dish. This quick stir-fry features extra-firm tofu and tender broccoli florets, providing a rich source of protein, fiber, and essential nutrients. Sesame oil adds a delightful flavor, while garlic, low-sodium soy sauce, and optional red pepper flakes enhance the taste. Sprinkled with sesame seeds, this dish offers a satisfying crunch. Low in calories and cholesterol-free, it supports cardiovascular health. Enjoy this flavorful and wholesome meal, perfect for a balanced diet.

Spaghetti Squash Primavera

Yield: 4 servings | **Prep time:** 15 minutes | **Cook time:** 45 minutes

- 1 medium spaghetti squash (about 3 pounds)
- 2 tablespoons olive oil
- 1 medium zucchini, diced
- 1 medium yellow bell pepper, diced
- 1 medium red bell pepper, diced
- 1 cup cherry tomatoes, halved
- 3 cloves garlic, minced
- Salt and pepper to taste
- 1/4 cup grated Parmesan cheese (optional)
- Fresh basil for garnish (optional)

Nutritional Information:

Approximately 180 calories,	4g protein,
25g carbohydrates,	8g fat,
0mg cholesterol,	5g fiber,
540mg potassium,	90mg sodium.

1. Preheat your oven to 400°F (200°C). Cut the spaghetti squash in half lengthwise and remove the seeds. Place the halves cut-side down on a baking sheet and bake for 40 minutes or until tender.
2. While the squash is baking, heat the olive oil in a large skillet over medium heat. Add the zucchini, yellow bell pepper, and red bell pepper. Sauté until softened, about 5-7 minutes.
3. Add the cherry tomatoes and garlic to the skillet. Cook for an additional 2-3 minutes. Season with salt and pepper to taste.
4. Once the squash is done, use a fork to scrape out the flesh into spaghetti-like strands. Add these to the skillet and toss to combine with the vegetables.
5. Serve warm, optionally sprinkled with grated Parmesan cheese and garnished with fresh basil.

Spaghetti Squash Primavera is a light and nutritious dish perfect for a heart-healthy diet. Roasted spaghetti squash is combined with sautéed zucchini, bell peppers, cherry tomatoes, and garlic, creating a colorful and flavorful meal. This dish is rich in vitamins, fiber, and antioxidants, supporting overall cardiovascular health. Low in calories and carbohydrates, it's a great alternative to traditional pasta. Optionally, sprinkle with grated Parmesan cheese and garnish with fresh basil for added flavor. Enjoy this wholesome and satisfying meal that's both delicious and beneficial for maintaining a healthy lifestyle.

Quinoa Pilaf with Sun-Dried Tomatoes and Olives

Yield: 4 servings | **Prep time:** 10 minutes | **Cook time:** 20 minutes

- 1 cup quinoa, rinsed and drained
- 2 cups low-sodium vegetable broth
- 1/2 cup sun-dried tomatoes, chopped
- 1/2 cup Kalamata olives, pitted and chopped
- 1 small red onion, finely chopped
- 2 cloves garlic, minced
- 1 tablespoon olive oil
- Salt and pepper to taste
- 2 tablespoons fresh basil, chopped (for garnish)

Nutritional Information:

Approximately 280 calories,	8g protein,
40g carbohydrates,	10g fat,
0mg cholesterol,	5g fiber,
450mg potassium,	300mg sodium.

1. Heat the olive oil in a medium saucepan over medium heat. Add the red onion and garlic, sautéing until the onion is translucent, about 3-5 minutes.
2. Add the quinoa to the saucepan and stir for a minute to toast the grains.
3. Pour in the vegetable broth, bring to a boil, then reduce the heat to low, cover, and simmer for about 15 minutes or until the quinoa is cooked and the liquid is absorbed.
4. Stir in the chopped sun-dried tomatoes and Kalamata olives, and season with salt and pepper to taste. Cook for an additional 2-3 minutes to warm the added ingredients.
5. Garnish with fresh basil before serving.

Quinoa Pilaf with Sun-Dried Tomatoes and Olives is a flavorful and heart-healthy dish. This pilaf combines quinoa, a nutrient-rich grain, with the savory flavors of sun-dried tomatoes and Kalamata olives. Sautéed red onion and garlic enhance the taste, while low-sodium vegetable broth keeps the dish light and healthy. High in protein, fiber, and essential nutrients, this pilaf supports cardiovascular health. Garnish with fresh basil for added freshness and aroma. Enjoy this delicious and wholesome meal as a perfect side or light main course.

Mediterranean Polenta Stacks

Yield: 4 servings | **Prep time:** 15 minutes | **Cook time:** 25 minutes

- **1 tube (18 oz) pre-cooked polenta, sliced into 1-inch rounds**
- **1 tablespoon olive oil**
- **1 cup cherry tomatoes, halved**
- **1 small zucchini, thinly sliced**
- **1/4 cup Kalamata olives, pitted and chopped**
- **1/4 cup feta cheese, crumbled (optional)**
- **1 teaspoon dried oregano**
- **Salt and pepper to taste**
- **2 tablespoons fresh basil, chopped for garnish**

Nutritional Information:

Approximately 190 calories,	*5g protein,*
30g carbohydrates,	*6g fat,*
0mg cholesterol,	*4g fiber,*
380mg potassium,	*220mg sodium.*

1. Preheat the oven to 400°F (200°C). Lightly brush both sides of the polenta slices with olive oil and place them on a baking sheet. Bake for 20 minutes, turning once halfway through, until they begin to crisp.
2. While the polenta is baking, heat the remaining olive oil in a skillet over medium heat. Add the cherry tomatoes, zucchini, and oregano. Cook for about 5 minutes, stirring occasionally, until the vegetables are tender.
3. Assemble the stacks by placing a slice of baked polenta on a plate, followed by a spoonful of the vegetable mixture, a sprinkle of olives, and a little feta cheese if using.
4. Return the stacks to the oven for an additional 5 minutes to warm through. Remove from oven and garnish with fresh basil before serving.

Mediterranean Polenta Stacks are a delightful and heart-healthy dish. Slices of pre-cooked polenta are baked until crispy, then topped with a savory mix of cherry tomatoes, zucchini, and Kalamata olives, seasoned with oregano. Optional crumbled feta cheese adds a creamy texture, while fresh basil provides a fragrant garnish. This dish is low in calories and rich in fiber and potassium, supporting cardiovascular health. With a balance of flavors and textures, these polenta stacks make for a satisfying and nutritious meal, perfect for a balanced diet.

Creamy Avocado Pesto Zoodles

Yield: 4 servings | **Prep time:** 15 minutes | **Cook time:** 5 minutes

For Avocado Pesto:
- **1 ripe avocado, peeled and pitted**
- **1 cup fresh basil leaves**
- **2 cloves garlic**
- **2 tablespoons lemon juice**
- **1/4 cup pine nuts**
- **Salt and pepper to taste**
- **2 tablespoons olive oil**

For Zoodles:
- **4 medium zucchinis, spiralized**
- **1 tablespoon olive oil**
- **Salt and pepper to taste**
- **Optional: cherry tomatoes and fresh basil for garnish**

1. Place the avocado, basil, garlic, lemon juice, pine nuts, salt, and pepper in a food processor. Process until smooth, then gradually add the olive oil while the machine is running. Set aside.
2. Heat a large skillet over medium heat and add 1 tablespoon of olive oil. Add the spiralized zucchini (zoodles) and sauté for about 2-3 minutes, just until they soften.
3. Remove the skillet from heat, then add the creamy avocado pesto and mix well to coat the zoodles.

4. Season with additional salt and pepper if needed, and garnish with cherry tomatoes and fresh basil if using.

Nutritional Information:
Approximately 350 calories,

8g protein,

20g carbohydrates,

28g fat,

8g fiber,

0mg cholesterol,

180mg sodium,

900mg potassium.

Creamy Avocado Pesto Zoodles is a nutritious and heart-healthy dish perfect for a light meal. Spiralized zucchini noodles are sautéed and tossed in a rich avocado pesto made from fresh basil, garlic, lemon juice, and pine nuts. This dish is packed with healthy fats, fiber, and vitamins, supporting cardiovascular health. The creamy avocado provides a satisfying texture, while the fresh basil and lemon juice add vibrant flavors. Garnish with cherry tomatoes and additional basil for extra freshness. Enjoy this delicious and wholesome meal that's both low in carbohydrates and high in essential nutrients.

Balsamic Glazed Tofu with Roasted Vegetables

Yield: 4 servings | **Prep time:** 20 minutes | **Cook time:** 40 minutes

- **1 block (14 ounces) firm tofu, drained and pressed**
- **2 tablespoons olive oil**
- **2 tablespoons balsamic vinegar**
- **2 teaspoons soy sauce, low sodium**
- **2 cloves garlic, minced**
- **1 large zucchini, cut into 1-inch pieces**
- **1 large red bell pepper, cut into 1-inch pieces**
- **1 medium red onion, cut into wedges**
- **1 teaspoon dried thyme**
- **Salt and pepper to taste**

Nutritional Information:
Approximately 210 calories,

12g protein,

18g carbohydrates,

10g fat,

3g fiber,

0mg cholesterol,

320mg sodium,

400mg potassium.

1. Preheat your oven to 400°F (200°C). Cut tofu into 1-inch cubes and place them in a mixing bowl. Add 1 tablespoon of olive oil, 1 tablespoon of balsamic vinegar, soy sauce, and minced garlic. Toss to coat and let marinate for 10 minutes.
2. While tofu is marinating, prepare the vegetables. In another mixing bowl, add zucchini, bell pepper, and red onion. Add the remaining 1 tablespoon of olive oil and dried thyme. Toss to coat.
3. Spread marinated tofu and prepared vegetables on a baking sheet in a single layer. Season with salt and pepper.
4. Roast in the preheated oven for 20 minutes. Flip tofu and vegetables and roast for another 20 minutes or until vegetables are tender and tofu is crispy.
5. Drizzle remaining 1 tablespoon of balsamic vinegar over the roasted tofu and vegetables before serving.

Balsamic Glazed Tofu with Roasted Vegetables is a hearty and heart-healthy meal. Firm tofu is marinated in a mixture of balsamic vinegar, low-sodium soy sauce, and garlic, then roasted alongside zucchini, red bell pepper, and red onion seasoned with thyme. This dish is packed with plant-based protein, fiber, and essential nutrients, supporting cardiovascular health. The balsamic glaze adds a rich, tangy flavor to the crispy tofu and tender vegetables. With its balanced mix of flavors and textures, this meal is both satisfying and nutritious, perfect for a wholesome dinner.

Grilled Eggplant and Zucchini Lasagna

Yield: 4 servings | **Prep time:** 25 minutes | **Cook time:** 40 minutes

- 1 large eggplant, sliced into 1/2-inch rounds
- 2 medium zucchinis, sliced lengthwise into 1/4-inch strips
- 1 tablespoon olive oil
- 2 cups low-fat ricotta cheese
- 1 cup tomato sauce (low-sodium)
- 1/2 cup grated Parmesan cheese
- 1 cup shredded mozzarella cheese (low-fat)
- 2 cloves garlic, minced
- 1 teaspoon dried oregano
- 1 teaspoon dried basil
- Salt and pepper to taste

Nutritional Information:
Approximately 320 calories,
20g protein,
25g carbohydrates,
16g fat,
7g fiber,
35mg cholesterol,
300mg sodium,
600mg potassium.

1. Preheat grill to medium-high heat. Lightly brush eggplant and zucchini slices with olive oil and sprinkle with salt and pepper. Grill for about 5 minutes per side or until tender and grill marks appear.
2. Preheat your oven to 375°F (190°C). In a mixing bowl, combine ricotta cheese, minced garlic, oregano, basil, and a pinch of salt and pepper. Mix well.
3. In a 9x13-inch baking dish, spread a layer of tomato sauce. Place a layer of grilled eggplant slices over the sauce. Spread half of the ricotta mixture over the eggplant and sprinkle with Parmesan and mozzarella cheese.
4. Add a layer of grilled zucchini slices on top of the cheese. Repeat the layers, ending with a layer of tomato sauce and a sprinkle of Parmesan and mozzarella cheese.
5. Cover the baking dish with aluminum foil and bake for 30 minutes. Remove foil and bake for an additional 10 minutes or until the cheese is melted and bubbly. Allow to cool slightly before serving.

Grilled Eggplant and Zucchini Lasagna is a delicious and heart-healthy twist on traditional lasagna. Layers of grilled eggplant and zucchini provide a rich source of fiber and antioxidants, while low-fat ricotta and mozzarella cheeses offer a creamy, protein-packed filling. Using low-sodium tomato sauce helps keep the sodium content in check. This dish is seasoned with garlic, oregano, and basil for a burst of Italian flavor. Baked until bubbly and golden, this lasagna is both nutritious and satisfying, making it a perfect choice for a balanced, heart-conscious meal.

Cauliflower Steaks with Chimichurri Sauce

Yield: 4 servings | **Prep time:** 20 minutes | **Cook time:** 30 minutes

For the Cauliflower Steaks:
- 2 medium heads cauliflower
- 2 tablespoons olive oil
- Salt and pepper to taste

For the Chimichurri Sauce:
- 1 cup fresh parsley, finely chopped
- 1/2 cup fresh cilantro, finely chopped
- 3 cloves garlic, minced
- Juice of 1 lemon
- 1/2 cup olive oil
- Salt and pepper to taste

1. Preheat the oven to 400°F (200°C). Line a baking sheet with parchment paper.
2. Cut the cauliflower heads into 1-inch thick steaks. You should get about 2-3 steaks per cauliflower head. Place the steaks on the prepared baking sheet, drizzle with olive oil, and season with salt and pepper.
3. Roast the cauliflower steaks in the preheated oven for 25-30 minutes, flipping halfway through, until they are tender and slightly golden.
4. While the cauliflower is roasting, prepare the chimichurri sauce. In a bowl, combine the parsley, cilantro, garlic, lemon juice, and olive oil. Season with salt and pepper to taste.
5. Serve the roasted cauliflower steaks topped with the chimichurri sauce.

Nutritional Information:

Approximately 350 calories,

6g protein,

20g carbohydrates,

28g fat,

7g fiber,

0mg cholesterol,

250mg sodium,

900mg potassium.

Cauliflower Steaks with Chimichurri Sauce is a delicious and heart-healthy dish. Thick cauliflower steaks are roasted to tender perfection, then topped with a vibrant chimichurri sauce made from fresh parsley, cilantro, garlic, lemon juice, and olive oil. This flavorful combination offers a nutritious meal rich in fiber, vitamins, and healthy fats. Low in carbohydrates and free from cholesterol, this dish supports cardiovascular health while delivering a satisfying and savory experience. Enjoy this plant-based entrée as a tasty and wholesome addition to your diet.

Tempeh Stir-Fry with Bell Peppers and Snap Peas

Yield: 4 servings | **Prep time:** 20 minutes | **Cook time:** 15 minutes

- **1 package (8 oz) tempeh, cut into cubes**
- **1 tablespoon olive oil**
- **1 red bell pepper, sliced**
- **1 yellow bell pepper, sliced**
- **1 cup snap peas, trimmed**
- **2 cloves garlic, minced**
- **1 tablespoon soy sauce (low-sodium)**
- **1 tablespoon hoisin sauce**
- **1 teaspoon ginger, minced**
- **Salt and pepper to taste**
- **Optional: 1 tablespoon sesame seeds for garnish**

1. In a large skillet or wok, heat the olive oil over medium-high heat. Add the tempeh cubes and cook until golden brown, about 5 minutes. Remove the tempeh and set it aside.
2. In the same skillet, add the garlic, bell peppers, and snap peas. Stir-fry for about 5 minutes, or until the vegetables are tender but still crisp.
3. Return the tempeh to the skillet and add the soy sauce, hoisin sauce, and minced ginger. Stir well to combine all the ingredients.
4. Season with salt and pepper to taste. If using, sprinkle sesame seeds over the top for garnish.

Nutritional Information:

Approximately 220 calories,	*14g protein,*
20g carbohydrates,	*10g fat,*
0mg cholesterol,	*4g fiber,*
420mg potassium,	*300mg sodium.*

Tempeh Stir-Fry with Bell Peppers and Snap Peas is a vibrant and heart-healthy dish. Cubed tempeh is cooked until golden brown and then stir-fried with crisp bell peppers and snap peas, adding a colorful array of vitamins and fiber. The dish is seasoned with garlic, ginger, low-sodium soy sauce, and hoisin sauce, providing a savory and slightly sweet flavor profile. Low in calories and rich in protein, this stir-fry supports cardiovascular health. Optional sesame seeds add a delightful crunch. Enjoy this nutritious and delicious meal, perfect for a balanced diet.

Vegetarian Taco Salad with Black Beans

Yield: 4 servings | **Prep time:** 15 minutes | **Cook time:** 10 minutes

- 1 can (15 ounces) black beans, drained and rinsed
- 1 tablespoon olive oil
- 1 small onion, finely chopped
- 1 clove garlic, minced
- 1 teaspoon ground cumin
- Salt and pepper to taste
- 4 cups romaine lettuce, chopped
- 1 cup cherry tomatoes, halved
- 1 avocado, diced
- 1 cup corn kernels, cooked
- 1/2 cup low-fat Greek yogurt
- Juice of 1 lime
- 1/4 cup fresh cilantro, chopped
- 1/2 cup low-fat shredded cheddar cheese (optional)

1. In a skillet over medium heat, add olive oil, onion, and garlic. Sauté until onion is translucent. Add black beans, cumin, salt, and pepper. Cook for about 5 minutes, stirring occasionally. Remove from heat and set aside.
2. In a large bowl, combine chopped lettuce, cherry tomatoes, avocado, and corn.
3. In a small bowl, mix low-fat Greek yogurt and lime juice to make the dressing.
4. Assemble the salad by layering the bean mixture over the lettuce mixture. Drizzle the dressing on top and garnish with chopped cilantro. If using, sprinkle shredded cheddar cheese on top.

Nutritional Information:

Approximately 350 calories,	*14g protein,*
45g carbohydrates,	*13g fat,*
5mg cholesterol,	*12g fiber,*
800mg potassium,	*300mg sodium.*

Vegetarian Taco Salad with Black Beans is a nutritious and heart-healthy meal. This vibrant salad features a base of chopped romaine lettuce topped with a flavorful mix of black beans seasoned with cumin, sautéed onions, and garlic. Cherry tomatoes, avocado, and corn add color and nutrients. A tangy dressing made from low-fat Greek yogurt and lime juice ties it all together, with fresh cilantro for extra freshness. Optional low-fat shredded cheddar cheese adds a tasty touch. This salad is packed with protein, fiber, and healthy fats, making it both delicious and satisfying.

Thai Vegetable Curry with Coconut Milk

Yield: 4 servings | **Prep time:** 15 minutes | **Cook time:** 20 minutes

- 1 tablespoon olive oil
- 1 small onion, diced
- 2 cloves garlic, minced
- 1 red bell pepper, sliced
- 1 zucchini, sliced
- 1 carrot, sliced
- 1 cup snap peas
- 1 can (13.5 oz) light coconut milk
- 2 tablespoons Thai red curry paste
- 1 teaspoon turmeric powder
- 1 teaspoon ground cumin
- Salt and pepper to taste
- 2 cups cooked brown rice (for serving)
- Fresh cilantro for garnish (optional)

1. Heat the olive oil in a large pan over medium heat. Add the onion and garlic and sauté until translucent, about 3 minutes.
2. Stir in the red curry paste, turmeric, and cumin until the onion and garlic are well-coated.
3. Add the sliced red bell pepper, zucchini, carrot, and snap peas to the pan. Stir for a couple of minutes.
4. Pour in the light coconut milk, bring to a simmer, and cook for 15 minutes or until the vegetables are tender. Adjust seasoning with salt and pepper.
5. Serve over cooked brown rice and garnish with fresh cilantro, if desired.

Nutritional Information:

Approximately 270 calories,	*6g protein,*
30g carbohydrates,	*15g fat,*
0mg cholesterol,	*4g fiber,*
500mg potassium,	*320mg sodium.*

Thai Vegetable Curry with Coconut Milk is a flavorful and heart-healthy dish. This curry features a medley of vegetables like red bell pepper, zucchini, carrot, and snap peas simmered in a creamy light coconut milk base, seasoned with Thai red curry paste, turmeric, and cumin. Served over cooked brown rice, it offers a balanced meal rich in fiber, vitamins, and healthy fats. Garnish with fresh cilantro for added freshness. This vibrant and nutritious curry is perfect for a delicious and satisfying meal that supports cardiovascular health. Enjoy this easy-to-make and delightful dish!

Curried Chickpea and Spinach Curry

Yield: 4 servings | **Prep time:** 15 minutes | **Cook time:** 30 minutes

- **2 cans (15 oz each) chickpeas, drained and rinsed**
- **1 tablespoon olive oil**
- **1 medium onion, finely chopped**
- **3 cloves garlic, minced**
- **1-inch piece of ginger, grated**
- **1 can (14 oz) coconut milk (low-fat)**
- **4 cups fresh spinach**
- **2 tablespoons curry powder**
- **1 teaspoon ground cumin**
- **Salt and pepper to taste**
- **2 tablespoons lemon juice**

1. Heat the olive oil in a large skillet over medium heat. Add the onion, garlic, and ginger. Sauté until the onion is translucent, about 5 minutes.
2. Stir in the curry powder, ground cumin, salt, and pepper. Cook for another 2 minutes to toast the spices.
3. Add the chickpeas and coconut milk to the skillet. Stir well and bring the mixture to a simmer. Cover and cook for 20 minutes.
4. Stir in the fresh spinach and cook until wilted, about 5 minutes.
5. Finish with lemon juice, stir well, and serve hot.

Nutritional Information:

Approximately 340 calories,	*14g protein,*
40g carbohydrates,	*12g fat,*
0mg cholesterol,	*12g fiber,*
720mg potassium,	*300mg sodium.*

Curried Chickpea and Spinach Curry is a flavorful and heart-healthy dish perfect for any meal. Packed with protein-rich chickpeas and nutrient-dense spinach, this curry is simmered in a creamy low-fat coconut milk base. Seasoned with aromatic curry powder, cumin, garlic, and ginger, it offers a rich and satisfying taste. A splash of lemon juice adds a refreshing finish. Low in fat and high in fiber, this curry supports cardiovascular health while providing essential vitamins and minerals. Enjoy this nutritious and delicious curry served hot for a wholesome dining experience.

Vegetable and Lentil Shepherd's Pie

Yield: 4 servings | **Prep time:** 20 minutes | **Cook time:** 45 minutes

- **2 cups cooked green lentils**
- **4 medium potatoes, peeled and cubed**
- **1/4 cup unsweetened almond milk**
- **1 tablespoon olive oil**
- **1 medium onion, diced**
- **2 cloves garlic, minced**
- **1 cup carrots, diced**
- **1 cup peas**
- **1 cup corn kernels**
- **1 tablespoon tomato paste**
- **2 teaspoons dried thyme**
- **Salt and pepper to taste**

Nutritional Information:

Approximately 350 calories,   *18g protein,*
60g carbohydrates,   *4g fat,*
0mg cholesterol,   *15g fiber,*
800mg potassium,   *300mg sodium*

1. Preheat your oven to 400°F (200°C). Boil the cubed potatoes in salted water until tender, approximately 15 minutes. Drain and mash them with the almond milk. Set aside.
2. In a large skillet, heat the olive oil over medium heat. Add the onion and garlic, sautéing until translucent. Add the carrots, peas, and corn, cooking until the vegetables are tender, about 10 minutes.
3. Stir in the cooked lentils, tomato paste, and thyme. Season with salt and pepper to taste.
4. Transfer the lentil and vegetable mixture into a baking dish. Evenly spread the mashed potatoes on top.
5. Bake for 25-30 minutes, or until the top is lightly golden. Allow to cool for a few minutes before serving.

Vegetable and Lentil Shepherd's Pie is a hearty and heart-healthy dish. This recipe features a flavorful mix of cooked green lentils, carrots, peas, and corn, seasoned with thyme and tomato paste. Topped with creamy mashed potatoes made with almond milk, it's baked to perfection with a golden crust. High in protein, fiber, and essential nutrients, this dish supports cardiovascular health and provides a satisfying meal. Low in fat and cholesterol-free, it's a nutritious and delicious option for a balanced diet. Enjoy this wholesome shepherd's pie as a comforting and nourishing dinner.

Red Lentil Dahl with Brown Rice

Yield: 4 servings | **Prep time:** 15 minutes | **Cook time:** 35 minutes

- **1 cup red lentils, rinsed and drained**
- **4 cups low-sodium vegetable broth**
- **1 cup brown rice**
- **1 tablespoon olive oil**
- **1 medium onion, finely chopped**
- **3 cloves garlic, minced**
- **1 tablespoon ginger, minced**
- **1 teaspoon ground cumin**
- **1 teaspoon ground coriander**
- **1/2 teaspoon turmeric**
- **1/2 teaspoon chili powder (optional, for heat)**
- **Salt and pepper to taste**
- **Fresh cilantro for garnish (optional)**

1. In a pot, bring 2 cups of water to a boil. Add the brown rice, reduce heat to low, cover, and simmer for 30-35 minutes or until rice is tender.
2. In a separate pot, add red lentils and vegetable broth. Bring to a boil, then reduce to a simmer. Cook for about 20 minutes or until lentils are tender.

3. While the lentils and rice are cooking, heat olive oil in a skillet over medium heat. Add the chopped onion, garlic, and ginger, sautéing until translucent.
4. Add ground cumin, coriander, turmeric, and chili powder to the skillet. Stir to combine and cook for another 2 minutes.
5. Once the lentils are done, drain any excess liquid and add them to the skillet. Stir well to combine all the ingredients. Season with salt and pepper to taste.

Nutritional Information:
Approximately 340 calories,
14g protein,
60g carbohydrates,
5g fat,
10g fiber,
0mg cholesterol,
200mg sodium,
400mg potassium.

Red Lentil Dahl with Brown Rice is a nutritious and heart-healthy meal. This dish features red lentils cooked in a flavorful mix of ground cumin, coriander, turmeric, garlic, and ginger, providing a rich source of protein and fiber. Paired with wholesome brown rice, it creates a satisfying and balanced meal. Low in fat and cholesterol-free, this dahl supports cardiovascular health while offering a warming, spiced flavor. Optionally garnish with fresh cilantro for added freshness. Enjoy this delicious, comforting dish that's perfect for a healthy and balanced diet.

Roasted Butternut Squash Risotto

Yield: 4 servings | **Prep time:** 20 minutes | **Cook time:** 40 minutes

- **1 medium butternut squash, peeled and diced (about 4 cups)**
- **1 tablespoon olive oil**
- **Salt and pepper to taste**
- **1 1/2 cups Arborio rice**
- **4 cups low-sodium vegetable broth, warmed**
- **1 medium onion, finely chopped**
- **2 cloves garlic, minced**
- **1/2 cup dry white wine (optional)**
- **1 teaspoon dried thyme**
- **1/2 teaspoon dried sage**
- **2 tablespoons nutritional yeast or grated Parmesan (optional)**

1. Preheat the oven to 400°F (200°C). Toss the butternut squash with olive oil, salt, and pepper. Spread on a baking sheet and roast for 20-25 minutes or until tender.
2. In a large saucepan, sauté the onion and garlic with a splash of water or broth until translucent, about 5 minutes.
3. Add the Arborio rice to the saucepan and stir for a minute to toast the rice. If using, pour in the white wine and cook until it's mostly evaporated.
4. Add the warmed vegetable broth, one cup at a time, stirring frequently. Wait until the liquid is mostly absorbed before adding the next cup.
5. Once the rice is tender, stir in the roasted butternut squash, dried thyme, dried sage, and optional nutritional yeast or Parmesan. Adjust seasoning with salt and pepper to taste.

Nutritional Information:
Approximately 380 calories,	*8g protein,*
75g carbohydrates,	*4g fat,*
0mg cholesterol,	*6g fiber,*
700mg potassium,	*220mg sodium.*

Roasted Butternut Squash Risotto is a delicious and heart-healthy dish. This creamy risotto combines roasted butternut squash with Arborio rice, creating a satisfying meal rich in fiber and essential nutrients. Sautéed onion and garlic add depth of flavor, while dried thyme and sage bring a warm, aromatic touch. Using low-sodium vegetable broth keeps the sodium content in check, supporting cardiovascular health. Optional nutritional yeast or Parmesan enhances the creamy texture without adding much fat. Enjoy this comforting risotto for a nutritious and flavorful meal perfect for a balanced diet.

Zucchini and Corn Fritters

Yield: 4 servings | **Prep time:** 20 minutes | **Cook time:** 15 minutes

- 2 medium zucchinis, grated
- 1 cup corn kernels (fresh or frozen)
- 1/4 cup chopped green onions
- 1/2 teaspoon salt
- 1/4 teaspoon black pepper
- 1/4 teaspoon paprika
- 1/2 cup whole wheat flour
- 1/4 cup cornmeal
- 2 eggs or egg substitute for vegan option
- 1 tablespoon olive oil for frying

1. Place the grated zucchini in a clean kitchen towel and squeeze out as much moisture as possible.
2. In a mixing bowl, combine the drained zucchini, corn kernels, and green onions. Add in the salt, black pepper, and paprika. Mix well.
3. Stir in the whole wheat flour and cornmeal. Beat the eggs and add them to the mixture, combining everything thoroughly.
4. Heat the olive oil in a non-stick skillet over medium heat. Drop spoonfuls of the mixture into the skillet and flatten slightly to form fritters. Cook for 3-4 minutes on each side or until golden brown.
5. Place the cooked fritters on a paper towel to remove excess oil, and serve immediately.

Nutritional Information:
Approximately 210 calories,
8g protein,
32g carbohydrates,
6g fat,
4g fiber,
90mg cholesterol (if using real eggs),
340mg sodium,
400mg potassium.

Zucchini and Corn Fritters are a tasty and heart-healthy dish. Grated zucchini and corn kernels are mixed with green onions, whole wheat flour, and cornmeal, then seasoned with paprika, salt, and pepper. These fritters are lightly fried in olive oil, creating a crispy exterior while maintaining a tender inside. High in fiber and essential nutrients, these fritters support cardiovascular health. For a vegan option, substitute the eggs with an egg substitute. Serve these golden-brown fritters immediately for a delicious, nutritious meal that's perfect for any occasion.

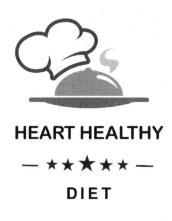

HEART HEALTHY

— ★★★★★ —

DIET

Chapter

12

Smoothie and Juice

Avocado and Mint Green Smoothie

Yield: 2 servings | **Prep time:** 7 minutes | **Cook time:** 0 minutes

- **1 medium avocado, peeled and pitted**
- **1/2 cup fresh mint leaves**
- **1 medium cucumber, peeled and sliced**
- **1 cup baby spinach leaves**
- **1 lime, juiced**
- **1 cup coconut water**
- **1 tablespoon chia seeds**
- **1 tablespoon honey or agave nectar (optional)**
- **Ice cubes (optional)**

Nutritional Information:

Approximately 220 calories,

24g carbohydrates,

0mg cholesterol,

4g protein,

14g fat,

9g fiber,

610mg potassium,

115mg sodium.

1. Place the avocado, mint leaves, cucumber, baby spinach, and lime juice into a blender.
2. Add the chia seeds, optional honey or agave nectar, and coconut water.
3. Blend on high speed until smooth and creamy. If the smoothie is too thick, add more coconut water or some ice cubes and blend again.
4. Taste and adjust sweetness, if needed, by adding more honey or agave nectar.
5. Pour into glasses and serve immediately.

Avocado and Mint Green Smoothie is a refreshing and heart-healthy drink. This smoothie combines creamy avocado with fresh mint leaves, cucumber, baby spinach, and lime juice, all blended with hydrating coconut water. Chia seeds add fiber and healthy fats, while optional honey or agave nectar provides a touch of sweetness. This nutrient-packed beverage supports cardiovascular health, digestion, and hydration. Blend until smooth and enjoy immediately for a revitalizing and creamy drink that's perfect for a healthy start to your day or a nourishing snack.

Kale and Pineapple Detox Smoothie

Yield: 2 servings | **Prep time:** 10 minutes | **Cook time:** 0 minutes

- 1 cup kale leaves, stems removed
- 1 cup pineapple chunks, fresh or frozen
- 1 banana, peeled
- 1/2 lemon, juiced
- 1 tablespoon chia seeds
- 1 tablespoon flax seeds
- 1 1/2 cups unsweetened almond milk or coconut water
- Ice cubes (optional)

Nutritional Information:

Approximately 180 calories,	5g protein,
35g carbohydrates,	4g fat,
0mg cholesterol,	7g fiber,
600mg potassium,	110mg sodium.

1. Place the kale, pineapple, banana, lemon juice, chia seeds, and flax seeds into a blender.
2. Add the almond milk or coconut water and blend until smooth. If the smoothie is too thick, you can add more liquid or some ice cubes and blend again.
3. Taste and adjust the sweetness or acidity by adding more banana or lemon juice, if needed.
4. Pour into glasses and serve immediately.

Kale and Pineapple Detox Smoothie is a refreshing and heart-healthy drink perfect for a nutritious boost. Combining kale and pineapple with banana, lemon juice, chia seeds, and flax seeds, this smoothie is rich in vitamins, fiber, and antioxidants. Unsweetened almond milk or coconut water adds hydration without extra calories. This smoothie supports cardiovascular health and digestion while offering a deliciously tropical flavor. Blend until smooth and enjoy immediately for a revitalizing and nutrient-packed beverage, perfect for starting your day or as a healthy snack.

Berry Antioxidant Blast Smoothie

Yield: 2 servings | **Prep time:** 5 minutes | **Cook time:** 0 minutes

- 1 cup mixed berries (strawberries, blueberries, raspberries, and blackberries), fresh or frozen
- 1 medium banana
- 1/2 cup Greek yogurt, non-fat
- 1/2 cup unsweetened almond milk
- 1 tablespoon chia seeds
- 1 tablespoon honey or agave nectar (optional)
- Ice cubes (optional)

Nutritional Information:

Approximately 180 calories,	8g protein,
32g carbohydrates,	3g fat,
0mg cholesterol,	6g fiber,
420mg potassium,	55mg sodium.

1. Place the mixed berries, banana, Greek yogurt, and almond milk into a blender.
2. Add the chia seeds and optional honey or agave nectar for sweetness.
3. Blend on high speed until smooth. If the smoothie is too thick, you can add more almond milk or some ice cubes and blend again.
4. Pour into glasses and serve immediately.

Berry Antioxidant Blast Smoothie is a delicious and heart-healthy drink, perfect for a quick and nutritious boost. This smoothie combines mixed berries, rich in antioxidants, with a banana, non-fat Greek yogurt, and unsweetened almond milk. Chia seeds add fiber and healthy fats, while optional honey or agave nectar provides natural sweetness. Blend until smooth and enjoy immediately for a refreshing and nutrient-packed beverage. This smoothie supports cardiovascular health, provides a good source of protein, and is low in fat, making it an ideal choice for a healthy snack or breakfast.

Chocolate Peanut Butter Protein Smoothie

Yield: 2 servings | **Prep time:** 5 minutes | **Cook time:** 0 minutes

- **1 cup unsweetened almond milk**
- **1 medium banana, frozen and sliced**
- **2 tablespoons unsweetened peanut butter**
- **1 tablespoon unsweetened cocoa powder**
- **1 scoop plant-based chocolate protein powder (about 20-25g)**
- **1 tablespoon chia seeds**
- **1 teaspoon vanilla extract**
- **Ice cubes (optional)**

Nutritional Information:

Approximately 260 calories,	*15g protein,*
22g carbohydrates,	*14g fat,*
0mg cholesterol,	*7g fiber,*
350mg potassium,	*190mg sodium.*

1. Place the unsweetened almond milk, frozen banana slices, unsweetened peanut butter, and unsweetened cocoa powder in a blender.
2. Add the plant-based chocolate protein powder, chia seeds, and vanilla extract to the blender.
3. Blend on high speed until smooth and creamy. If the smoothie is too thick, you can add a few ice cubes or additional almond milk and blend again.
4. Once blended, taste and adjust sweetness or flavor as needed.
5. Pour into glasses and serve immediately.

Chocolate Peanut Butter Protein Smoothie is a delicious and heart-healthy drink, perfect for a post-workout boost or a nutritious snack. This smoothie combines unsweetened almond milk, frozen banana, unsweetened peanut butter, and cocoa powder for a rich and creamy base. Plant-based chocolate protein powder and chia seeds add protein and fiber, supporting muscle recovery and heart health. Vanilla extract enhances the flavor. Blend until smooth and adjust the thickness with ice cubes or additional almond milk if needed. Enjoy this satisfying and nutritious smoothie immediately for a delicious treat.

Tropical Turmeric Smoothie

Yield: 2 servings | **Prep time:** 7 minutes | **Cook time:** 0 minutes

- **1 cup coconut water**
- **1/2 cup frozen mango chunks**
- **1/2 cup frozen pineapple chunks**
- **1 medium banana**
- **1/2 teaspoon ground turmeric**
- **1/2 teaspoon ground ginger**
- **1 tablespoon chia seeds**
- **1 tablespoon flaxseeds**
- **A pinch of black pepper (to enhance turmeric absorption)**

Nutritional Information:

Approximately 180 calories,	*3g protein,*
38g carbohydrates,	*3g fat,*
0mg cholesterol,	*7g fiber,*
700mg potassium,	*90mg sodium.*

1. Add the coconut water, frozen mango chunks, frozen pineapple chunks, and banana to the blender.
2. Sprinkle in the ground turmeric, ground ginger, chia seeds, flaxseeds, and a pinch of black pepper.
3. Blend on high until smooth and creamy. If the mixture is too thick, add a little more coconut water and blend again.
4. Taste the smoothie and adjust the seasoning if necessary.
5. Pour into glasses and serve immediately.

Tropical Turmeric Smoothie is a refreshing and heart-healthy drink that combines the vibrant flavors of mango, pineapple, and banana with the anti-inflammatory benefits of turmeric and ginger. Chia seeds and flaxseeds add fiber and omega-3 fatty acids, while coconut water provides hydration. A pinch of black pepper enhances turmeric absorption. Blend until smooth and creamy, adjusting the consistency with additional coconut water if needed. Enjoy this nutritious and delicious smoothie immediately for a tropical treat that supports cardiovascular health and overall wellness.

Blueberry and Spinach Powerhouse Smoothie

Yield: 2 servings | **Prep time:** 5 minutes | **Cook time:** 0 minutes

- 1 cup almond milk (unsweetened)
- 1 cup fresh blueberries
- 1 cup baby spinach
- 1 medium banana
- 1 tablespoon chia seeds
- 1 tablespoon hemp seeds
- 1 teaspoon honey or maple syrup (optional for sweetness)
- A handful of ice cubes

Nutritional Information:

Approximately 160 calories, 5g protein, 28g carbohydrates, 4g fat, 0mg cholesterol, 6g fiber, 400mg potassium, 125mg sodium

1. In a blender, add the almond milk, fresh blueberries, baby spinach, and banana.
2. Add in the chia seeds, hemp seeds, and honey or maple syrup if using.
3. Toss in a handful of ice cubes for added chill.
4. Blend on high speed until the smoothie is smooth and creamy.
5. Taste and adjust sweetness, if needed, before pouring into glasses and serving immediately.

Blueberry and Spinach Powerhouse Smoothie is a nutrient-rich and heart-healthy drink, perfect for a quick energy boost. This smoothie blends fresh blueberries, baby spinach, and banana with unsweetened almond milk, providing a mix of antioxidants, fiber, and essential vitamins. Chia seeds and hemp seeds add protein and healthy fats, while optional honey or maple syrup offers a touch of sweetness. Ice cubes give it a refreshing chill. Blend until smooth and creamy, then enjoy immediately for a delicious and revitalizing beverage that supports overall health and well-being.

Ginger and Carrot Immunity Smoothie

Yield: 2 servings | **Prep time:** 10 minutes | **Cook time:** 0 minutes

- 1 cup carrot juice (freshly squeezed or store-bought, unsweetened)
- 1 medium banana
- 1-inch piece of fresh ginger, peeled
- 1/2 cup coconut water
- 1 medium orange, peeled and segmented
- 1 tablespoon flaxseeds
- A pinch of ground turmeric
- Ice cubes (optional)

Nutritional Information:

Approximately 140 calories, 3g protein, 32g carbohydrates, 1g fat, 0mg cholesterol, 4g fiber, 500mg potassium, 100mg sodium.

1. Add the carrot juice, banana, ginger, and coconut water to a blender.
2. Add the orange segments, flaxseeds, and ground turmeric.
3. If using ice cubes, add them to the blender.
4. Blend on high speed until everything is smooth and well combined.
5. Pour into glasses and serve immediately.

Ginger and Carrot Immunity Smoothie is a refreshing and heart-healthy drink designed to boost your immune system. Combining freshly squeezed carrot juice with banana, fresh ginger, and coconut water, this smoothie is rich in vitamins and antioxidants. Orange segments add a zesty citrus flavor, while flaxseeds provide fiber and omega-3 fatty acids. A pinch of turmeric enhances the anti-inflammatory properties. Blend until smooth and creamy, adding ice cubes for extra chill if desired. Enjoy this nutritious smoothie immediately to support overall health and well-being.

Apple and Oat Breakfast Smoothie

Yield: 2 servings | **Prep time:** 10 minutes | **Cook time:** 0 minutes

- **1 large apple, cored and sliced**
- **1/2 cup rolled oats**
- **1 cup unsweetened almond milk**
- **1 medium banana**
- **1 tablespoon chia seeds**
- **1 teaspoon cinnamon**
- **1/2 teaspoon vanilla extract**
- **Ice cubes (optional)**

1. Add the apple slices, rolled oats, and almond milk to a blender. Allow the mixture to sit for about 5 minutes to soften the oats.
2. Add the banana, chia seeds, cinnamon, and vanilla extract to the blender.
3. If using ice cubes, add them to the blender.
4. Blend on high speed until smooth and creamy.
5. Pour into glasses and serve immediately.

Nutritional Information:

Approximately 220 calories,   5g protein,
40g carbohydrates,   5g fat,
0mg cholesterol,   8g fiber,
350mg potassium,   90mg sodium.

Apple and Oat Breakfast Smoothie is a nutritious and heart-healthy way to start your day. This smoothie blends apple slices, rolled oats, and unsweetened almond milk, providing a fiber-rich base. Adding banana, chia seeds, cinnamon, and vanilla extract enhances the flavor and nutritional value, offering a boost of vitamins, antioxidants, and omega-3 fatty acids. Allowing the oats to soften ensures a smooth texture. Blend until creamy and enjoy immediately for a satisfying and energizing breakfast that supports cardiovascular health and overall well-being.

Peaches and Cream Vegan Smoothie

Yield: 2 servings | **Prep time:** 10 minutes | **Cook time:** 0 minutes

- **2 cups frozen peach slices**
- **1 cup unsweetened almond milk**
- **1 medium banana, frozen**
- **1 tablespoon chia seeds**
- **1 teaspoon vanilla extract**
- **2 tablespoons rolled oats**
- **Ice cubes (optional)**

Nutritional Information:

Approximately 200 calories,   4g protein,
45g carbohydrates,   4g fat,
0mg cholesterol,   7g fiber,
400mg potassium,   80mg sodium.

1. Place the frozen peach slices, almond milk, and frozen banana in a blender.
2. Add chia seeds, vanilla extract, and rolled oats to the blender.
3. If using ice cubes, add them to the blender for extra thickness.
4. Blend on high until the smoothie is creamy and smooth.
5. Pour the smoothie into glasses and serve immediately.

Peaches and Cream Vegan Smoothie is a delicious and heart-healthy drink perfect for any time of day. This smoothie blends frozen peach slices, unsweetened almond milk, and a frozen banana for a creamy base. Adding chia seeds, vanilla extract, and rolled oats provides fiber, healthy fats, and a boost of nutrients. Blend until smooth and creamy, adding ice cubes if desired for extra thickness. Enjoy this refreshing and nutritious smoothie immediately for a satisfying, dairy-free treat that supports cardiovascular health and overall well-being.

Mango and Chia Seed Hydration Smoothie

Yield: 2 servings | **Prep time:** 10 minutes | **Cook time:** 0 minutes

- **1 large ripe mango, peeled and pitted (about 1.5 cups of mango chunks)**
- **1 cup coconut water**
- **1 tablespoon chia seeds**
- **1/2 lime, juiced**
- **1/2 cup ice cubes (optional)**
- **1 teaspoon honey or agave syrup (optional, for added sweetness)**

Nutritional Information:

Approximately 150 calories,	*2g protein,*
35g carbohydrates,	*2g fat,*
0mg cholesterol,	*5g fiber,*
400mg potassium,	*95mg sodium.*

1. Start by soaking the chia seeds in the coconut water for about 5-10 minutes until they form a gel-like consistency.
2. Add the mango chunks to a blender.
3. Add the chia seed and coconut water mixture, lime juice, and ice cubes if using.
4. Blend until smooth, adding honey or agave syrup if needed for extra sweetness.
5. Pour into glasses and serve immediately.

Mango and Chia Seed Hydration Smoothie is a refreshing and heart-healthy drink, perfect for staying hydrated. This smoothie combines ripe mango chunks with coconut water, offering natural sweetness and essential electrolytes. Chia seeds add fiber and omega-3 fatty acids, while a splash of lime juice enhances the flavor with a tangy twist. Blend until smooth, adding ice cubes for extra chill and optional honey or agave syrup for added sweetness. Enjoy this hydrating and nutritious smoothie immediately, ideal for boosting your overall health and well-being.

Beet and Pomegranate Heart Juice

Yield: 2 servings | **Prep time:** 15 minutes | **Cook time:** 0 minutes

- **1 medium beet, peeled and cut into chunks**
- **1 pomegranate, seeds removed (about 1 cup of seeds)**
- **1 large carrot, peeled and cut into chunks**
- **1 apple, cored and sliced**
- **1/2 lemon, peeled**
- **1 inch fresh ginger, peeled**

Nutritional Information:

Approximately 130 calories,	*2g protein,*
32g carbohydrates,	*1g fat,*
0mg cholesterol,	*6g fiber,*
400mg potassium,	*70mg sodium.*

1. Prepare all the fruits and vegetables by peeling and cutting them into sizes that will easily fit into your juicer.
2. Start juicing the beet chunks, followed by the pomegranate seeds, carrot, apple, lemon, and ginger.
3. Once everything has been juiced, give the mixture a good stir to combine all the flavors.
4. Pour the juice through a strainer into glasses to remove any remaining pulp (optional).
5. Serve immediately or refrigerate for later use.

Beet and Pomegranate Heart Juice is a nutrient-rich and heart-healthy drink, perfect for boosting cardiovascular health. This juice combines the earthy sweetness of beets with the vibrant flavors of pomegranate seeds, carrot, apple, lemon, and fresh ginger. Packed with antioxidants, vitamins, and minerals, this refreshing juice supports overall heart health and vitality. Simply juice all the ingredients, stir well, and strain if desired to remove pulp. Enjoy immediately or refrigerate for later use. This delicious juice is a great way to nourish your body and support a healthy lifestyle.

Orange and Carrot Glow Juice

Yield: 4 servings | **Prep time:** 10 minutes | **Cook time:** 0 minutes

- **4 large oranges, peeled and quartered**
- **6 medium carrots, peeled and cut into chunks**
- **1-inch piece of fresh ginger, peeled**
- **1 lemon, peeled and quartered**
- **A pinch of turmeric powder (optional)**

Nutritional Information:

Approximately 110 calories,

2g protein,

26g carbohydrates,

1g fat,

4g fiber,

0mg cholesterol,

60mg sodium,

450mg potassium.

1. Prepare all the fruits and vegetables by peeling and cutting them into sizes that will easily fit into your juicer.
2. Begin juicing the oranges, followed by the carrots, ginger, and lemon. Add a pinch of turmeric powder if desired.
3. Stir the juice well to combine all the flavors.
4. Pour the juice through a strainer into a pitcher or directly into glasses to remove any remaining pulp (optional).
5. Serve immediately, or refrigerate and consume within 24 hours for best quality.

Orange and Carrot Glow Juice is a vibrant and nutritious drink perfect for boosting your skin's radiance and overall health. This refreshing juice combines the natural sweetness of oranges and carrots with the zesty kick of lemon and ginger. A pinch of turmeric powder can be added for its anti-inflammatory benefits. Packed with vitamins, antioxidants, and essential nutrients, this juice supports your immune system and promotes a healthy glow. Simply juice the ingredients, stir well, and strain if desired. Enjoy immediately or refrigerate for up to 24 hours for the best quality.

Ginger and Lemon Wellness Shot

Yield: 4 servings | **Prep time:** 5 minutes | **Cook time:** 0 minutes

- **1 large lemon, peeled**
- **2-inch piece of fresh ginger, peeled**
- **1 tablespoon turmeric powder**
- **A pinch of black pepper**
- **1 cup of cold water**

Nutritional Information:

Approximately 15 calories,

0.4g protein,

4g carbohydrates,

0.1g fat,

0.8g fiber,

0mg cholesterol,

2mg sodium,

60mg potassium.

1. Peel the lemon and ginger. Cut them into small pieces that will fit easily into your blender.
2. Place the lemon, ginger, turmeric powder, and a pinch of black pepper into the blender.
3. Add 1 cup of cold water and blend on high speed until you get a smooth mixture.
4. Using a fine-mesh strainer or cheesecloth, strain the mixture into a jar or directly into shot glasses, discarding the pulp.
5. Consume immediately, or store in the refrigerator for up to 48 hours. Shake well before use.

Ginger and Lemon Wellness Shot is a potent and heart-healthy drink designed to boost your immune system and overall wellness. Combining fresh lemon and ginger with turmeric powder and a pinch of black pepper enhances the anti-inflammatory benefits and absorption of nutrients. This shot is packed with antioxidants and vitamins, providing a quick and refreshing boost to your daily routine. Blend all ingredients with cold water, strain, and consume immediately for maximum benefits, or refrigerate for up to 48 hours, shaking well before each use. Enjoy this invigorating wellness shot as part of your healthy lifestyle.

HEART HEALTHY

— ★★★★★ —

DIET

Chapter

13

Dessert

Avocado Chocolate Mousse

Yield: 4 servings | **Prep time:** 10 minutes | **Cook time:** 0 minutes

- **2 ripe avocados, peeled and pitted**
- **1/4 cup unsweetened cocoa powder**
- **1/4 cup almond milk (or any unsweetened non-dairy milk)**
- **2 tablespoons pure maple syrup**
- **1 teaspoon vanilla extract**
- **A pinch of sea salt**
- **Fresh berries for garnish (optional)**

Nutritional Information:
Approximately 210 calories,   *3g protein,*
19g carbohydrates,   *15g fat,*
0mg cholesterol,   *7g fiber,*
450mg potassium,   *80mg sodium*

1. Cut the avocados in half, remove the pit, and scoop the flesh into a blender or food processor.
2. Add unsweetened cocoa powder, almond milk, maple syrup, vanilla extract, and a pinch of sea salt to the blender or food processor.
3. Blend until smooth, stopping occasionally to scrape down the sides of the blender or food processor with a spatula.
4. Taste and adjust sweetness by adding more maple syrup if needed. Blend again to incorporate any additional sweetener.
5. Spoon the mousse into dessert cups or bowls, and garnish with fresh berries if desired. Serve immediately or refrigerate until ready to serve.

Avocado Chocolate Mousse is a rich and creamy dessert that's both heart-healthy and delicious. Made with ripe avocados, unsweetened cocoa powder, almond milk, maple syrup, and vanilla extract, this mousse offers a luscious texture without dairy. A pinch of sea salt enhances the flavors, while optional fresh berries add a burst of freshness. Blend until smooth and serve in dessert cups, either immediately or chilled. With approximately 210 calories per serving, this mousse is a nutritious treat high in healthy fats, fiber, and antioxidants. Enjoy this guilt-free dessert that satisfies chocolate cravings and supports overall wellness.

Banana and Walnut Bread

Yield: 6 servings | **Prep time:** 15 minutes | **Cook time:** 60 minutes

- **3 ripe bananas, mashed**
- **1/4 cup olive oil**
- **1/4 cup unsweetened applesauce**
- **1/4 cup pure maple syrup**
- **1 teaspoon vanilla extract**
- **1 1/2 cups whole-wheat flour**
- **1 teaspoon baking soda**
- **1/2 teaspoon cinnamon**
- **1/4 teaspoon salt**
- **1/2 cup chopped walnuts**

Nutritional Information:

Approximately 350 calories,	*6g protein,*
50g carbohydrates,	*15g fat,*
0mg cholesterol,	*6g fiber,*
400mg potassium,	*250mg sodium.*

1. Preheat your oven to 350°F (175°C). Line a 9x5-inch loaf pan with parchment paper or lightly grease it.
2. In a mixing bowl, combine mashed bananas, olive oil, applesauce, maple syrup, and vanilla extract. Mix until smooth.
3. In another bowl, whisk together whole-wheat flour, baking soda, cinnamon, and salt.
4. Add the dry ingredients to the wet ingredients and mix just until combined. Fold in the chopped walnuts.
5. Pour the batter into the prepared loaf pan and bake for 60 minutes or until a toothpick inserted into the center comes out clean.

Banana and Walnut Bread is a wholesome and heart-healthy treat perfect for breakfast or a snack. This recipe combines ripe bananas, olive oil, unsweetened applesauce, and pure maple syrup for natural sweetness and moisture. Whole-wheat flour, baking soda, cinnamon, and salt create a nutritious base, while chopped walnuts add a delightful crunch and healthy fats. Bake until golden brown and enjoy a slice that's rich in fiber and essential nutrients. With approximately 350 calories per serving, this bread supports cardiovascular health and provides lasting energy throughout the day.

Blueberry Oatmeal Crumble Bars

Yield: 6 servings | **Prep time:** 20 minutes | **Cook time:** 40 minutes

- **2 cups fresh blueberries**
- **1 tablespoon lemon juice**
- **1 tablespoon cornstarch**
- **2 cups old-fashioned oats**
- **1 cup whole-wheat flour**
- **1/2 cup pure maple syrup**
- **1/4 cup unsweetened applesauce**
- **1/4 cup olive oil**
- **1 teaspoon cinnamon**
- **1/4 teaspoon salt**

Nutritional Information:

Approximately 270 calories,	*4g protein,*
45g carbohydrates,	*9g fat,*
0mg cholesterol,	*5g fiber,*
180mg potassium,	*100mg sodium.*

1. Preheat the oven to 350°F (175°C). Line an 8x8-inch baking pan with parchment paper.
2. In a small bowl, mix blueberries, lemon juice, and cornstarch. Set aside.
3. In a large bowl, combine oats, whole-wheat flour, maple syrup, applesauce, olive oil, cinnamon, and salt. Mix until well combined.
4. Press 2/3 of the oat mixture into the bottom of the prepared baking pan. Spread the blueberry mixture evenly over the oat layer.
5. Crumble the remaining oat mixture over the blueberries and gently press down. Bake for 40 minutes, or until the top is lightly golden.

Blueberry Oatmeal Crumble Bars are a delicious and heart-healthy treat, perfect for breakfast or a snack. Fresh blueberries are combined with lemon juice and cornstarch to create a sweet and tangy filling. The crust and crumble topping are made from old-fashioned oats, whole-wheat flour, pure maple syrup, unsweetened applesauce, and olive oil, with a hint of cinnamon and a pinch of salt for flavor. These bars are baked until golden brown and packed with fiber, antioxidants, and essential nutrients. Enjoy these nutritious and tasty bars, each with approximately 270 calories per serving.

Cinnamon-Spiced Baked Apples

Yield: 4 servings | Prep time: 15 minutes | Cook time: 45 minutes

- **4 medium-sized apples, cored and sliced**
- **2 tablespoons pure maple syrup**
- **1 teaspoon ground cinnamon**
- **1/4 teaspoon ground nutmeg**
- **1/4 cup chopped walnuts**
- **1/4 cup old-fashioned oats**
- **1 tablespoon olive oil**

Nutritional Information:

Approximately 210 calories,	*2g protein,*
40g carbohydrates,	*7g fat,*
0mg cholesterol,	*5g fiber,*
250mg potassium,	*5mg sodium.*

1. Preheat your oven to 350°F (175°C). Grease a baking dish lightly with olive oil or line it with parchment paper.
2. In a bowl, toss the apple slices with maple syrup, cinnamon, and nutmeg.
3. Place the spiced apple slices in the prepared baking dish.
4. In a separate bowl, mix the chopped walnuts, oats, and olive oil. Sprinkle this mixture over the apples.
5. Bake for 45 minutes, or until the apples are tender and the topping is slightly crispy.

Cinnamon-Spiced Baked Apples are a comforting and heart-healthy dessert perfect for any occasion. Sliced apples are tossed with pure maple syrup, ground cinnamon, and nutmeg, then topped with a mixture of chopped walnuts, old-fashioned oats, and olive oil. Baked until tender and slightly crispy, these apples offer a delightful blend of flavors and textures. Rich in fiber and essential nutrients, this dessert supports cardiovascular health. Enjoy these warm, spiced apples for a delicious and nutritious treat with approximately 210 calories per serving.

Dark Chocolate and Almond Bark

Yield: 6 servings | Prep time: 10 minutes | Cook time: 5 minutes

- **8 oz dark chocolate (70% or higher cocoa content)**
- **1/2 cup whole almonds, roasted**
- **1/4 cup dried cranberries or cherries (optional)**
- **1/4 teaspoon sea salt**
- **1 teaspoon orange zest (optional)**

Nutritional Information:

Approximately 210 calories,
4g protein,
16g carbohydrates,
16g fat,
3g fiber,
0mg cholesterol,
100mg sodium,
230mg potassium.

1. Line a baking sheet with parchment paper or a silicone baking mat.
2. Melt the dark chocolate in a microwave-safe bowl at 20-second intervals, stirring after each interval, or use a double boiler.
3. Once the chocolate is melted, stir in the almonds, dried cranberries or cherries, and orange zest, if using.
4. Pour the chocolate mixture onto the prepared baking sheet, spreading it out with a spatula into a layer of your desired thickness. Sprinkle sea salt on top.
5. Allow it to cool in the refrigerator for at least 1 hour. Once solid, break it into pieces.

Dark Chocolate and Almond Bark is a simple yet indulgent treat that's heart-healthy and delicious. Made with high-quality dark chocolate (70% or higher cocoa content), roasted whole almonds, and optional dried cranberries or cherries, this bark is rich in antioxidants, fiber, and healthy fats. A touch of sea salt enhances the flavors, while optional orange zest adds a hint of citrus. Melt and mix the ingredients, spread on a baking sheet, and cool in the refrigerator until solid. Enjoy this nutritious and satisfying snack with approximately 210 calories per serving.

Vegan Lemon Sorbet

Yield: 4 servings | **Prep time:** 10 minutes | **Cook time:** 0 minutes (additional freezing time required)

- **1 cup lemon juice, freshly squeezed**
- **1 cup water**
- **1/2 cup agave syrup or maple syrup**
- **Zest of 1 lemon**
- **A pinch of sea salt**

Nutritional Information:
 Approximately 100 calories,
 0g protein,
 26g carbohydrates,
 0g fat,
 0g fiber,
 0mg cholesterol,
 20mg sodium,
 50mg potassium.

1. In a medium bowl, whisk together lemon juice, water, agave syrup, lemon zest, and a pinch of sea salt until well combined.
2. Pour the mixture into a shallow dish and place it in the freezer.
3. After 1 hour, use a fork to break up any ice crystals. Return to the freezer.
4. Repeat step 3 every 30 minutes until the sorbet is fully frozen and has a smooth texture, about 3-4 hours total.
5. Before serving, allow the sorbet to sit at room temperature for 5 minutes to make it easier to scoop. Serve immediately.

Vegan Lemon Sorbet is a refreshing and heart-healthy dessert perfect for warm days. Made with freshly squeezed lemon juice, water, agave or maple syrup, lemon zest, and a pinch of sea salt, this sorbet offers a burst of citrus flavor with a smooth, icy texture. Simply mix the ingredients, freeze, and periodically break up the ice crystals until fully frozen. This light and zesty treat is low in calories and free of cholesterol, making it an ideal option for a guilt-free dessert. Enjoy this delightful sorbet with approximately 100 calories per serving.

No-Bake Peanut Butter Energy Bites

Yield: 6 servings (approximately 18 energy bites) | **Prep time:** 15 minutes | **Cook time:** 0 minutes

- **1 cup old-fashioned oats**
- **1/2 cup natural peanut butter**
- **1/3 cup honey or maple syrup**
- **1/2 cup ground flaxseed**
- **1/2 cup mini dark chocolate chips**
- **1 teaspoon vanilla extract**
- **A pinch of sea salt**

Nutritional Information:
 Approximately 200 calories,   6g protein,
 22g carbohydrates,   11g fat,
 0mg cholesterol,   4g fiber,
 150mg potassium,   50mg sodium.

1. In a large mixing bowl, combine the old-fashioned oats, natural peanut butter, honey or maple syrup, ground flaxseed, mini dark chocolate chips, vanilla extract, and a pinch of sea salt.
2. Mix all ingredients until well combined.
3. Using your hands, form the mixture into 1-inch balls and place them on a tray lined with parchment paper.
4. Place the tray in the refrigerator for at least 30 minutes to allow the energy bites to firm up.
5. Store in an airtight container in the refrigerator for up to one week.

No-Bake Peanut Butter Energy Bites are a quick and nutritious snack perfect for on-the-go fuel. Made with old-fashioned oats, natural peanut butter, honey or maple syrup, ground flaxseed, mini dark chocolate chips, vanilla extract, and a pinch of sea salt, these energy bites offer a balanced mix of protein, fiber, and healthy fats. Simply mix the ingredients, form into balls, and refrigerate to firm up. These bites are ideal for a mid-day snack or pre-workout boost, providing approximately 200 calories per serving. Enjoy their delicious, wholesome flavor and energy-boosting benefits!

Gluten-Free Carrot Cake with Cashew Frosting

Yield: 6 servings | **Prep time:** 30 minutes | **Cook time:** 30 minutes

For the Cake:
- **2 cups gluten-free all-purpose flour**
- **1 teaspoon baking powder**
- **1/2 teaspoon baking soda**
- **1 teaspoon cinnamon**
- **1/2 teaspoon nutmeg**
- **1/4 teaspoon salt**
- **1/2 cup unsweetened applesauce**
- **1/4 cup coconut oil, melted**
- **1/2 cup maple syrup or honey**
- **2 cups grated carrots**
- **1/2 cup crushed pineapple, drained**
- **1 teaspoon vanilla extract**

For the Cashew Frosting:
- **1 cup cashews, soaked for at least 4 hours and drained**
- **1/4 cup coconut cream**
- **2 tablespoons lemon juice**
- **2 tablespoons maple syrup or honey**
- **1 teaspoon vanilla extract**

1. Preheat the oven to 350°F (175°C). Grease an 8-inch round cake pan and line it with parchment paper.
2. In a large bowl, mix together the gluten-free flour, baking powder, baking soda, cinnamon, nutmeg, and salt. In a separate bowl, combine the applesauce, melted coconut oil, maple syrup, grated carrots, crushed pineapple, and vanilla extract.
3. Fold the wet ingredients into the dry ingredients until just combined. Pour the batter into the prepared cake pan.
4. Bake for 30 minutes or until a toothpick inserted into the center of the cake comes out clean. Let the cake cool completely.
5. While the cake is cooling, prepare the cashew frosting by blending all frosting ingredients in a high-speed blender until smooth. Spread the frosting over the cooled cake.

Nutritional Information:

Approximately 420 calories,	7g protein,
62g carbohydrates,	18g fat,
5g fiber,	0mg cholesterol,
420mg potassium,	220mg sodium.

Gluten-Free Carrot Cake with Cashew Frosting is a delightful and healthy dessert option that is perfect for any occasion. This moist and flavorful cake is made with gluten-free all-purpose flour, grated carrots, crushed pineapple, and a blend of warm spices like cinnamon and nutmeg. Sweetened with maple syrup or honey and applesauce, it's a wholesome treat. The creamy cashew frosting, made with soaked cashews, coconut cream, lemon juice, and vanilla extract, adds a rich and smooth finish. Each serving contains approximately 420 calories, making it a nutritious and satisfying indulgence.

Strawberry and Basil Frozen Yogurt

Yield: 4 servings | **Prep time:** 15 minutes | **Cook time:** 0 minutes (plus freezing time)

- **3 cups fresh strawberries, hulled**
- **1 cup low-fat Greek yogurt**
- **1/3 cup honey or maple syrup**
- **1/4 cup fresh basil leaves**
- **1 teaspoon vanilla extract**
- **A pinch of salt**

Nutritional Information:

Approximately 160 calories,	5g protein,
30g carbohydrates,	1g fat,
5mg cholesterol,	3g fiber,
200mg potassium,	50mg sodium.

1. In a blender, combine strawberries, Greek yogurt, honey, basil leaves, vanilla extract, and a pinch of salt. Blend until smooth.
2. Pour the mixture into an ice cream maker and churn according to the manufacturer's instructions until it reaches a soft-serve consistency.
3. Transfer the churned mixture to an airtight container and freeze for at least 2 hours to firm up before serving.
4. Before serving, let the frozen yogurt sit out at room temperature for 5-10 minutes to soften slightly.

Strawberry and Basil Frozen Yogurt is a refreshing and healthy treat perfect for warm days. Combining fresh strawberries, low-fat Greek yogurt, honey or maple syrup, basil leaves, and a hint of vanilla, this frozen delight offers a unique blend of flavors. The mixture is churned in an ice cream maker to achieve a creamy consistency and then frozen to firm up. With approximately 160 calories per serving, this dessert is rich in protein, fiber, and essential nutrients, making it a guilt-free indulgence. Enjoy this delicious and nutritious frozen yogurt as a delightful way to cool down and satisfy your sweet tooth.

Matcha and Almond Cookies

Yield: 6 servings (about 18 cookies) | **Prep time:** 20 minutes | **Cook time:** 10 minutes

- **1 cup almond flour**
- **2 tablespoons matcha (green tea) powder**
- **1/4 cup coconut oil, melted**
- **1/4 cup honey or maple syrup**
- **1 teaspoon vanilla extract**
- **1/4 teaspoon baking soda**
- **A pinch of salt**
- **1/4 cup chopped almonds**

Nutritional Information:

Approximately 160 calories,	3g protein,
14g carbohydrates,	10g fat,
0mg cholesterol,	2g fiber,
80mg potassium,	60mg sodium.

1. Preheat your oven to 350°F (175°C). Line a baking sheet with parchment paper.
2. In a mixing bowl, combine almond flour, matcha powder, baking soda, and a pinch of salt.
3. In another bowl, mix together the melted coconut oil, honey, and vanilla extract.
4. Combine the wet and dry ingredients, then fold in the chopped almonds.
5. Scoop out small portions of the dough and place them on the prepared baking sheet. Flatten them slightly with a fork. Bake for 10 minutes or until the edges turn golden brown.

Matcha and Almond Cookies are a delightful and healthy treat, combining the earthy flavor of matcha with the nutty richness of almonds. Made with almond flour, melted coconut oil, honey or maple syrup, and a hint of vanilla, these cookies are both gluten-free and dairy-free. Chopped almonds add a satisfying crunch. With only 10 minutes of baking time, these cookies are quick and easy to prepare. Each cookie offers approximately 160 calories, making them a nutritious and tasty snack that's perfect for any time of the day. Enjoy these vibrant green cookies as a wholesome indulgence.

Coconut and Berry Chia Pudding

Yield: 4 servings | **Prep time:** 15 minutes | **Cook time:** 0 minutes (Chill time: 2-4 hours)

- **1/4 cup chia seeds**
- **1 cup unsweetened coconut milk**
- **1/2 teaspoon vanilla extract**
- **1 tablespoon maple syrup or honey (optional)**
- **1 cup mixed berries (blueberries, raspberries, and strawberries)**
- **1/4 cup shredded unsweetened coconut**
- **A pinch of sea salt**

Nutritional Information:

Approximately 210 calories,	4g protein,
18g carbohydrates,	15g fat,
0mg cholesterol,	8g fiber,
250mg potassium,	90mg sodium.

1. In a bowl, combine the chia seeds, unsweetened coconut milk, vanilla extract, maple syrup or honey, and a pinch of sea salt. Stir well to avoid clumping.
2. Cover the bowl with plastic wrap or a lid and place it in the refrigerator for at least 2-4 hours, or overnight for best results.
3. Before serving, give the pudding a good stir to distribute the chia seeds evenly. If the mixture is too thick, you can add a little more coconut milk to reach your desired consistency.
4. In serving bowls, layer the chia pudding with mixed berries and top with shredded coconut.

Coconut and Berry Chia Pudding is a delicious and heart-healthy dessert or breakfast option. This creamy pudding combines chia seeds, unsweetened coconut milk, vanilla extract, and optional maple syrup or honey for natural sweetness. The mixture is chilled until it thickens, then layered with mixed berries and topped with shredded coconut. Packed with fiber, healthy fats, and antioxidants, this pudding is both satisfying and nutritious. Enjoy this easy-to-make treat with approximately 210 calories per serving, perfect for a healthy start to your day or a light dessert.

Raspberry Almond Tartlets

Yield: 6 servings | **Prep time:** 20 minutes | **Cook time:** 15 minutes

- **1 cup almond flour**
- **2 tablespoons coconut oil, melted**
- **2 tablespoons maple syrup**
- **1/4 teaspoon almond extract**
- **1/4 teaspoon salt**
- **1/2 cup raspberry jam (low sugar or no sugar added)**
- **1/2 cup fresh raspberries**
- **2 tablespoons sliced almonds**
- **Cooking spray or parchment paper for lining**

Nutritional Information:

Approximately 190 calories,	*4g protein,*
20g carbohydrates,	*11g fat,*
0mg cholesterol,	*3g fiber,*
70mg potassium,	*40mg sodium.*

1. Preheat the oven to 350°F (175°C). Grease a mini muffin tin or line it with parchment paper.
2. In a bowl, combine the almond flour, melted coconut oil, maple syrup, almond extract, and salt. Mix until a dough forms.
3. Press about 1 tablespoon of the almond mixture into each muffin cup, creating a small tart shell.
4. Fill each tart shell with about 1-2 teaspoons of raspberry jam, top with a fresh raspberry, and sprinkle with sliced almonds.
5. Bake in the preheated oven for 15 minutes or until the edges are golden brown. Allow to cool before serving.

Raspberry Almond Tartlets are a delightful and heart-healthy dessert, perfect for any occasion. These mini tartlets feature a crust made from almond flour, melted coconut oil, maple syrup, and almond extract, providing a rich, nutty base. Filled with raspberry jam and topped with a fresh raspberry and sliced almonds, they offer a perfect balance of sweetness and texture. Baked to golden perfection, these tartlets are as pleasing to the eye as they are to the palate. Each serving contains approximately 190 calories, making them a nutritious and satisfying treat. Enjoy these elegant tartlets as a delicious and healthy dessert option.

Maple-Roasted Peaches

Yield: 4 servings | **Prep time:** 10 minutes | **Cook time:** 25 minutes

- **4 ripe peaches, halved and pitted**
- **2 tablespoons pure maple syrup**
- **1 teaspoon vanilla extract**
- **1/2 teaspoon ground cinnamon**
- **1/4 teaspoon ground nutmeg**
- **A pinch of salt**
- **Cooking spray or parchment paper for lining**

Nutritional Information:

Approximately 90 calories,	*1g protein,*
23g carbohydrates,	*0g fat,*
0mg cholesterol,	*2g fiber,*
285mg potassium,	*10mg sodium.*

1. Preheat the oven to 400°F (200°C). Line a baking sheet with parchment paper or lightly spray with cooking spray.
2. In a small bowl, mix together the maple syrup, vanilla extract, cinnamon, and nutmeg.
3. Place the peach halves, cut-side up, on the prepared baking sheet. Drizzle the maple syrup mixture over the peaches.
4. Roast in the preheated oven for 25 minutes or until the peaches are tender and the edges are slightly caramelized.

Maple-Roasted Peaches are a simple yet elegant dessert, perfect for highlighting the natural sweetness of ripe peaches. Halved peaches are drizzled with a delightful mixture of pure maple syrup, vanilla extract, ground cinnamon, and nutmeg, then roasted until tender and slightly caramelized. This dessert is not only delicious but also low in calories, with approximately 90 calories per serving. Enjoy these warm, fragrant peaches on their own or with a dollop of yogurt or a scoop of ice cream for an extra treat. This heart-healthy dessert is both satisfying and nutritious, perfect for any occasion.

HEART HEALTHY

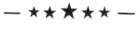

DIET

Chapter
14

Snack

Almond and Cranberry Trail Mix

Yield: 4 servings | **Prep time:** 5 minutes | **Cook time:** 0 minutes

- **1 cup raw almonds**
- **1/2 cup unsweetened dried cranberries**
- **1/4 cup pumpkin seeds (pepitas)**
- **1/4 cup unsweetened shredded coconut**
- **Optional: A pinch of sea salt**

Nutritional Information:

Approximately 330 calories,	9g protein,
25g carbohydrates,	23g fat,
0mg cholesterol,	7g fiber,
350mg potassium,	20mg sodium.

1. In a large mixing bowl, combine the raw almonds, unsweetened dried cranberries, pumpkin seeds, and shredded coconut.
2. If using, add a pinch of sea salt for flavor. Toss everything together until well mixed.
3. Divide the mixture into individual portion-sized containers or snack bags.
4. Store the trail mix in an airtight container to keep it fresh for up to 2 weeks.

Almond and Cranberry Trail Mix is a quick and nutritious snack perfect for on-the-go. Combining raw almonds, unsweetened dried cranberries, pumpkin seeds, and shredded coconut, this mix offers a balanced blend of protein, healthy fats, and fiber. Simply mix all the ingredients in a bowl, optionally adding a pinch of sea salt for extra flavor. Store the mixture in individual portion-sized containers or snack bags for convenience. This trail mix can be kept fresh in an airtight container for up to two weeks, providing a healthy and satisfying snack with approximately 330 calories per serving.

Spiced Chickpea Crunchies

Yield: 4 servings | **Prep time:** 10 minutes | **Cook time:** 40 minutes

- **2 cans (15 oz each) chickpeas, drained and rinsed**
- **1 tablespoon olive oil**
- **1 teaspoon smoked paprika**
- **1/2 teaspoon garlic powder**
- **1/2 teaspoon ground cumin**
- **1/4 teaspoon cayenne pepper (optional for heat)**
- **Salt to taste**

Nutritional Information:

Approximately 180 calories,	*9g protein,*
24g carbohydrates,	*6g fat,*
0mg cholesterol,	*7g fiber,*
280mg potassium,	*480mg sodium.*

1. Preheat your oven to 400°F (200°C). Line a baking sheet with parchment paper.
2. Drain and rinse the chickpeas, then pat them dry with a paper towel.
3. In a large bowl, toss the chickpeas with olive oil and spices until well coated.
4. Spread the chickpeas in a single layer on the prepared baking sheet.
5. Roast for 35-40 minutes, stirring every 10 minutes, until the chickpeas are crispy.

Spiced Chickpea Crunchies are a heart-healthy snack perfect for a diet focused on cardiovascular wellness. Chickpeas are rich in fiber and plant-based protein, which help lower cholesterol levels and maintain healthy blood sugar levels. The olive oil provides heart-healthy monounsaturated fats, while the spices, including smoked paprika and cumin, add anti-inflammatory benefits. Low in saturated fat and cholesterol-free, this crunchy snack is ideal for supporting heart health and overall well-being. Enjoy these flavorful, crispy chickpeas as a nutritious alternative to traditional snacks.

Veggie Hummus Dip Cups

Yield: 4 servings | **Prep time:** 15 minutes | **Cook time:** 0 minutes

- **1 cup hummus (store-bought or homemade)**
- **1 cup cherry tomatoes, halved**
- **1 cup baby carrots**
- **1 cup cucumber slices**
- **1 cup bell pepper slices**
- **1 tablespoon olive oil (optional)**
- **1 teaspoon paprika (optional for garnish)**
- **Salt and pepper to taste**

Nutritional Information:

Approximately 220 calories,	*8g protein,*
25g carbohydrates,	*11g fat,*
0mg cholesterol,	*8g fiber,*
400mg potassium,	*360mg sodium.*

1. Arrange 4 small serving cups or bowls on a platter.
2. Spoon about 1/4 cup of hummus into each cup.
3. Arrange the cherry tomatoes, baby carrots, cucumber slices, and bell pepper slices around the hummus in each cup.
4. If using, drizzle a little olive oil over the hummus and sprinkle with paprika, salt, and pepper for extra flavor.

Veggie Hummus Dip Cups are a heart-healthy, nutrient-dense snack perfect for a diet focused on cardiovascular wellness. The hummus provides plant-based protein and fiber, essential for maintaining healthy cholesterol levels and supporting digestive health. Fresh vegetables like cherry tomatoes, baby carrots, cucumber, and bell pepper are packed with vitamins, minerals, and antioxidants that contribute to heart health by reducing inflammation and blood pressure. Low in saturated fat and cholesterol-free, these vibrant dip cups make a delicious and wholesome snack option for promoting a healthy heart.

Olive and Walnut Tapenade on Whole-Grain Toast

Yield: 4 servings | **Prep time:** 10 minutes | **Cook time:** 5 minutes

- 1 cup pitted Kalamata olives
- 1/2 cup walnuts
- 2 cloves garlic, peeled
- 1 tablespoon capers, drained
- Zest of 1 lemon
- Juice of 1/2 lemon
- 1/4 cup extra-virgin olive oil
- 4 slices of whole-grain toast
- Fresh parsley for garnish (optional)

Nutritional Information:

Approximately 280 calories,   5g protein,
16g carbohydrates,   23g fat,
0mg cholesterol,   3g fiber,
180mg potassium,   760mg sodium.

1. In a food processor, combine the Kalamata olives, walnuts, garlic, capers, lemon zest, and lemon juice. Pulse until coarsely chopped.
2. While the food processor is running, slowly add the extra-virgin olive oil until the mixture reaches a spreadable consistency.
3. Toast the whole-grain bread slices until they are crispy and golden brown.
4. Generously spread the olive and walnut tapenade onto each slice of toast. Garnish with fresh parsley if desired.

Veggie Hummus Dip Cups are a heart-healthy, nutrient-dense snack perfect for a diet focused on cardiovascular wellness. The hummus provides plant-based protein and fiber, essential for maintaining healthy cholesterol levels and supporting digestive health. Fresh vegetables like cherry tomatoes, baby carrots, cucumber, and bell pepper are packed with vitamins, minerals, and antioxidants that contribute to heart health by reducing inflammation and blood pressure. Low in saturated fat and cholesterol-free, these vibrant dip cups make a delicious and wholesome snack option for promoting a healthy heart.

Apple Slices with Almond Butter Drizzle

Yield: 4 servings | **Prep time:** 10 minutes | **Cook time:** 0 minutes

- 2 large apples, sliced into thin rounds
- 1/2 cup almond butter
- 1 tablespoon honey
- 1/4 teaspoon ground cinnamon
- A pinch of sea salt
- 2 tablespoons chia seeds (optional for garnish)

Nutritional Information:

Approximately 220 calories,   5g protein,
25g carbohydrates,   13g fat,
0mg cholesterol,   5g fiber,
200mg potassium,   80mg sodium.

1. Wash and slice the apples into thin rounds, removing the core if desired.
2. In a small bowl, mix almond butter, honey, ground cinnamon, and a pinch of sea salt until well combined.
3. Arrange the apple slices on a serving plate.
4. Drizzle the almond butter mixture over the apple slices, using a spoon or a piping bag.
5. Optionally, sprinkle chia seeds over the apple slices for added texture and nutrition.

Apple Slices with Almond Butter Drizzle is a heart-healthy snack ideal for a diet focused on cardiovascular wellness. Apples provide soluble fiber, which helps lower cholesterol levels and promote healthy digestion. Almond butter, rich in monounsaturated fats, aids in maintaining good cholesterol and reducing bad cholesterol. The addition of honey and cinnamon not only enhances flavor but also offers antioxidant properties. Sprinkling chia seeds adds omega-3 fatty acids and fiber, supporting heart health and overall nutrition. This snack is a tasty and nutritious way to promote a healthy heart.

Roasted Sweet Potato Rounds

Yield: 4 servings | **Prep time:** 10 minutes | **Cook time:** 25 minutes

- **2 large sweet potatoes, scrubbed and sliced into 1/2-inch rounds**
- **2 tablespoons olive oil**
- **1 teaspoon smoked paprika**
- **1/2 teaspoon garlic powder**
- **Salt and pepper to taste**
- **Fresh parsley for garnish (optional)**

Nutritional Information:

Approximately 160 calories,	*2g protein,*
27g carbohydrates,	*5g fat,*
0mg cholesterol,	*4g fiber,*
450mg potassium,	*80mg sodium.*

1. Preheat the oven to 400°F (200°C). Line a baking sheet with parchment paper.
2. In a large bowl, toss the sweet potato rounds with olive oil, smoked paprika, garlic powder, salt, and pepper until well coated.
3. Arrange the coated sweet potato rounds in a single layer on the prepared baking sheet.
4. Roast in the preheated oven for 25 minutes or until the sweet potatoes are tender and lightly browned, flipping halfway through cooking.
5. Remove from oven and optionally garnish with fresh parsley before serving.

Roasted Sweet Potato Rounds are a nutritious and heart-friendly snack, perfect for a heart-healthy diet. Sweet potatoes are rich in dietary fiber, vitamins A and C, and potassium, all of which contribute to cardiovascular health by helping to regulate blood pressure and reduce inflammation. The use of olive oil, a source of healthy monounsaturated fats, aids in lowering bad cholesterol levels. Smoked paprika and garlic powder add a flavorful touch without adding extra calories or sodium. Garnishing with fresh parsley provides additional antioxidants, making this dish both delicious and beneficial for your heart.

Zucchini Pizza Bites

Yield: 4 servings | **Prep time:** 15 minutes | **Cook time:** 10 minutes

- **2 medium zucchinis, sliced into 1/2-inch rounds**
- **1 cup marinara sauce (low-sodium, if possible)**
- **1 cup shredded mozzarella cheese (part-skim)**
- **1/2 cup mini turkey pepperoni slices (optional)**
- **1 tablespoon olive oil**
- **1/2 teaspoon dried oregano**
- **1/2 teaspoon dried basil**

Nutritional Information:

Approximately 160 calories,	*9g protein,*
10g carbohydrates,	*9g fat,*
20mg cholesterol,	*2g fiber,*
400mg potassium,	*320mg sodium.*

1. Preheat the oven to 375°F (190°C). Line a baking sheet with parchment paper.
2. Brush each zucchini slice lightly with olive oil and place them on the baking sheet.
3. Spoon a small amount of marinara sauce onto each zucchini slice, followed by a sprinkle of mozzarella cheese, a piece of turkey pepperoni (if using), and a sprinkle of dried herbs.
4. Bake for about 10 minutes or until the cheese is melted and bubbly, and the zucchini is tender.
5. Remove from the oven and allow to cool for a couple of minutes before serving.

Zucchini Pizza Bites are a heart-healthy and delicious alternative to traditional pizza, perfect for a heart-conscious diet. The zucchini base provides a low-calorie, nutrient-rich foundation packed with vitamins A and C, which support cardiovascular health. Using part-skim mozzarella cheese and mini turkey pepperoni helps reduce saturated fat and cholesterol intake. Additionally, the use of low-sodium marinara sauce and olive oil ensures that these pizza bites are lower in sodium and contain healthy monounsaturated fats, contributing to better heart health. Enjoy these bites guilt-free for a tasty and nutritious snack.

Sundried Tomato and Basil Pinwheels

Yield: 4 servings | **Prep time:** 20 minutes | **Cook time:** 0 minutes

- **1 whole-grain tortilla (10-inch)**
- **4 oz low-fat cream cheese, softened**
- **1/2 cup sundried tomatoes, chopped**
- **1/4 cup fresh basil leaves, finely chopped**
- **1 tablespoon olive oil**
- **Salt and pepper to taste**

Nutritional Information:
Approximately 160 calories,   6g protein,
20g carbohydrates,   7g fat,
4g fiber,
10mg cholesterol,
220mg sodium,
300mg potassium.

1. Lay the whole-grain tortilla flat on a clean surface.
2. In a small bowl, mix the softened low-fat cream cheese and olive oil until smooth. Spread this mixture evenly over the tortilla.
3. Sprinkle the chopped sundried tomatoes and fresh basil leaves over the cream cheese layer. Season with a pinch of salt and pepper, if desired.
4. Roll up the tortilla tightly, then slice into 1-inch pinwheels.
5. Arrange the pinwheels on a serving platter and serve immediately or cover and refrigerate until ready to serve.

Sundried Tomato and Basil Pinwheels are a perfect addition to a heart-healthy diet, offering a delicious and nutritious snack option. These pinwheels feature whole-grain tortillas, providing essential fiber that supports heart health by lowering cholesterol levels. The low-fat cream cheese helps keep saturated fat in check, while the sundried tomatoes and fresh basil add a burst of flavor and beneficial antioxidants. Olive oil contributes healthy monounsaturated fats, which are known to improve heart health. These pinwheels are easy to prepare and make for a light, satisfying snack or appetizer.

Baked Parmesan Zucchini Fries

Yield: 4 servings | **Prep time:** 15 minutes | **Cook time:** 25 minutes

- **2 medium zucchinis, cut into fries**
- **1/2 cup grated Parmesan cheese**
- **1/4 cup almond flour**
- **1 teaspoon garlic powder**
- **1/2 teaspoon paprika**
- **Salt and pepper to taste**
- **1 large egg, beaten**
- **Cooking spray or olive oil for greasing**

Nutritional Information:
Approximately 130 calories,   8g protein,
10g carbohydrates,   7g fat,
40mg cholesterol,   3g fiber,
360mg potassium,   220mg sodium.

1. Preheat your oven to 425°F (220°C). Line a baking sheet with parchment paper and lightly grease it with cooking spray or olive oil.
2. In a shallow bowl, combine the grated Parmesan, almond flour, garlic powder, and paprika. Add salt and pepper to taste.
3. Dip each zucchini fry into the beaten egg, making sure it's fully coated, and then roll it in the Parmesan mixture. Place the coated zucchini fries on the prepared baking sheet.
4. Bake for 25 minutes, or until the fries are golden brown and crisp.
5. Serve immediately with your favorite dipping sauce.

Baked Parmesan Zucchini Fries are a heart-healthy alternative to traditional fries, packed with nutrients and flavor. These fries use almond flour and Parmesan cheese for a crispy coating, providing protein and healthy fats without excess carbohydrates. Zucchini is rich in vitamins and minerals, including potassium, which helps maintain healthy blood pressure. The use of garlic powder and paprika adds a burst of flavor while keeping sodium levels in check. Baking instead of frying ensures lower calorie and fat content, making these fries a guilt-free, delicious snack or side dish for those on a heart-healthy diet.

Chia Seed and Berry Yogurt Parfait

Yield: 4 servings | **Prep time:** 15 minutes | **Cook time:** 0 minutes

- **1 cup low-fat Greek yogurt**
- **2 tablespoons chia seeds**
- **1 cup mixed berries (strawberries, blueberries, raspberries)**
- **1 tablespoon honey or maple syrup (optional)**
- **1/4 cup granola (optional)**
- **A dash of vanilla extract (optional)**

Nutritional Information:

Approximately 120 calories,	*10g protein,*
18g carbohydrates,	*2g fat,*
5mg cholesterol,	*6g fiber,*
120mg potassium,	*40mg sodium.*

1. In a bowl, mix the low-fat Greek yogurt with the chia seeds. If you're using vanilla extract or sweeteners like honey, add them to the yogurt mixture and stir well.
2. In serving glasses or jars, layer the yogurt-chia mixture at the bottom.
3. Add a layer of mixed berries on top of the yogurt-chia mixture.
4. If you're using granola, sprinkle it over the berries for an extra crunch.
5. Repeat the layers until the glasses are filled, ending with a layer of berries on top. Serve immediately or refrigerate for later use.

Chia Seed and Berry Yogurt Parfait is a heart-healthy breakfast or snack option that's rich in protein and fiber. Low-fat Greek yogurt provides a creamy base packed with protein, supporting muscle health and keeping you full longer. Chia seeds are high in omega-3 fatty acids, which are known for their heart-protective properties. Mixed berries add a burst of antioxidants, vitamins, and fiber, promoting cardiovascular health. The optional addition of granola adds a satisfying crunch and extra fiber. This parfait is low in fat and sodium, making it a delicious and nutritious choice for maintaining a healthy heart.

Crispy Kale Chips with Sea Salt

Yield: 4 servings | **Prep time:** 10 minutes | **Cook time:** 12 minutes

- **1 large bunch of kale, washed, dried, and torn into bite-sized pieces**
- **1 tablespoon olive oil**
- **1/2 teaspoon sea salt (or to taste)**

Nutritional Information:

Approximately 60 calories,	*2g protein,*
8g carbohydrates,	*3g fat,*
0mg cholesterol,	*1g fiber,*
330mg potassium,	*290mg sodium.*

1. Preheat the oven to 350°F (175°C). Line a baking sheet with parchment paper.
2. In a large bowl, toss the kale pieces with olive oil until they are evenly coated.
3. Spread the kale in a single layer on the prepared baking sheet. Try not to overlap the kale pieces to ensure they get crispy.
4. Sprinkle the sea salt evenly over the kale.
5. Bake for 10-12 minutes, or until the edges of the kale are browned but not burnt. Keep a close eye on them, as they can burn quickly.

Crispy Kale Chips with Sea Salt are an excellent, heart-healthy snack option, ideal for a heart-conscious diet. Kale is a powerhouse of nutrients, rich in vitamins A, C, and K, as well as antioxidants that help reduce oxidative stress and inflammation, which are key contributors to heart disease. The use of olive oil adds beneficial monounsaturated fats, which can help lower bad cholesterol levels. With just a light sprinkle of sea salt, these chips offer a satisfying crunch without the excess sodium found in conventional snacks. Enjoy these guilt-free chips for a nutrient-dense, heart-healthy treat.

HEART HEALTHY

— ★★★★★ —

DIET

Chapter

15

Herbal Teas

Turmeric and Ginger Anti-Inflammatory Tea

Yield: 4 servings | **Prep time:** 5 minutes | **Cook time:** 10 minutes

- **1 tablespoon turmeric powder**
- **1 tablespoon ginger root, freshly grated**
- **4 cups of water**
- **1 lemon, juiced**
- **Optional: 1 tablespoon of honey or stevia for sweetness**

Nutritional Information:
Approximately 10 calories,
0g protein,
2g carbohydrates,
0g fat,
0g fiber,
0mg cholesterol,
10mg sodium,
20mg potassium.

1. **Boil Water:** In a medium-sized pot, bring 4 cups of water to a boil.
2. **Prepare Ingredients:** While the water is heating, grate the ginger root and measure out the turmeric powder.
3. **Steep:** Once the water is boiling, add the turmeric powder and grated ginger to the pot. Reduce the heat to low and let simmer for 7-10 minutes.
4. **Strain and Add Lemon:** Strain the liquid into mugs or a teapot, discarding the steeped ginger. Add the lemon juice to the strained tea.
5. **Sweeten and Serve:** If desired, add honey or stevia to sweeten and stir well before serving.

Turmeric and Ginger Anti-Inflammatory Tea is a powerful blend aimed at reducing inflammation and promoting heart health. Turmeric is renowned for its anti-inflammatory properties, thanks to curcumin, which helps protect against heart disease. Ginger aids in digestion and also has anti-inflammatory effects. This tea is infused with lemon juice for a boost of vitamin C and added flavor. Sweeten with honey or stevia for a touch of natural sweetness. Enjoy this soothing tea regularly to support a healthy heart and reduce inflammation.

Soothing Lavender and Chamomile Blend

Yield: 4 servings | **Prep time:** 5 minutes | **Cook time:** 10 minutes

- **2 tablespoons dried lavender flowers**
- **2 tablespoons dried chamomile flowers**
- **4 cups of water**
- **Optional: 1 tablespoon of honey or stevia for sweetness**

Nutritional Information:

Approximately 2 calories,
0.5g carbohydrates,
0mg cholesterol,
10mg potassium,
0g protein,
0g fat,
0g fiber,
10mg sodium.

1. **Boil Water:** In a medium-sized pot, bring 4 cups of water to a boil.
2. **Prepare Herbs:** While the water is heating, measure out the dried lavender and chamomile flowers.
3. **Steep:** Once the water is boiling, add the herbs to the pot and remove from heat. Cover and let steep for 7-10 minutes.
4. **Strain and Serve:** Strain the liquid into mugs or a teapot, discarding the steeped herbs. If desired, sweeten with honey or stevia.

The Soothing Lavender and Chamomile Blend is a calming herbal infusion perfect for heart health. Lavender and chamomile are renowned for their relaxing properties, helping to reduce stress and promote restful sleep, both crucial for maintaining cardiovascular well-being. This gentle, caffeine-free blend can be enjoyed any time of day. Adding a touch of honey or stevia enhances its natural sweetness without significantly impacting its low-calorie profile. This soothing drink provides a serene and heart-friendly way to unwind and support overall wellness.

Peppermint and Lemon Digestive Tea

Yield: 4 servings | **Prep time:** 5 minutes | **Cook time:** 10 minutes

- **2 tablespoons dried peppermint leaves**
- **1 organic lemon, thinly sliced**
- **4 cups of water**
- **Optional: 1 tablespoon of honey or stevia for sweetness**

Nutritional Information:

Approximately 5 calories,
0g protein,
1g carbohydrates,
0g fat,
0g fiber,
0mg cholesterol,
8mg sodium,
15mg potassium.

1. **Boil Water:** In a medium-sized pot, bring 4 cups of water to a boil.
2. **Prepare Ingredients:** While the water is heating, measure out the dried peppermint leaves and thinly slice the lemon.
3. **Steep:** Once the water is boiling, add the peppermint leaves and lemon slices to the pot. Remove from heat, cover, and let steep for 7-10 minutes.
4. **Strain and Serve:** Strain the liquid into mugs or a teapot, discarding the steeped herbs and lemon slices. If desired, sweeten with honey or stevia.

The Peppermint and Lemon Digestive Tea is a refreshing blend designed to support heart health and aid digestion. Peppermint is known for its ability to soothe the digestive tract and reduce bloating, while lemon adds a burst of vitamin C and antioxidants, promoting overall cardiovascular health. This tea is easy to prepare, low in calories, and can be sweetened with honey or stevia for added flavor without significantly increasing calorie intake. Enjoy this soothing tea anytime to help maintain a healthy heart and digestive system.

Rosehip and Hibiscus Vitamin Boost Tea

Yield: 4 servings | **Prep time:** 5 minutes | **Cook time:** 10 minutes

- **4 cups water**
- **2 tablespoons dried rosehip**
- **2 tablespoons dried hibiscus flowers**
- **1 lemon, sliced (optional for added flavor)**
- **Optional: 1 tablespoon of honey or stevia for sweetness**

Nutritional Information:
Approximately 5 calories,
0g protein,
1g carbohydrates,
0g fat,
1g fiber,
0mg cholesterol,
10mg sodium,
15mg potassium.

1. **Boil Water:** In a medium-sized pot, bring 4 cups of water to a boil.
2. **Add Ingredients:** Once the water is boiling, add the dried rosehip and hibiscus flowers to the pot.
3. **Steep:** Reduce heat to low, cover, and let the tea steep for about 8-10 minutes.
4. **Strain and Serve:** Strain the liquid into mugs or a teapot, discarding the steeped rosehip and hibiscus. Add optional lemon slices for added flavor.
5. **Sweeten:** If desired, add honey or stevia to sweeten before serving.

Rosehip and Hibiscus Vitamin Boost Tea is a refreshing and health-enhancing beverage perfect for supporting heart health. Both rosehip and hibiscus are rich in antioxidants and vitamin C, which can help boost the immune system and promote cardiovascular health. Hibiscus is known for its ability to lower blood pressure and cholesterol levels, while rosehip provides anti-inflammatory benefits. Enjoy this vibrant tea hot or iced, optionally sweetened with honey or stevia, and with a hint of lemon for added zest and flavor.

Green Tea with Fresh Mint Leaves

Yield: 4 servings | **Prep time:** 5 minutes | **Cook time:** 5 minutes

- **4 cups water**
- **4 green tea bags or 4 teaspoons loose-leaf green tea**
- **1 handful fresh mint leaves (about 10-15 leaves)**
- **Optional: lemon slices for garnish**
- **Optional: honey or stevia for sweetness**

Nutritional Information:
Approximately 2 calories,
0g protein,
0g carbohydrates,
0g fat,
0g fiber,
0mg cholesterol,
0mg sodium,
20mg potassium.

1. **Boil Water:** In a pot, bring 4 cups of water to a rolling boil.
2. **Prepare Mint Leaves:** While waiting for the water to boil, rinse and pat dry the mint leaves.
3. **Steep Tea and Mint:** Once the water is boiling, turn off the heat, add the green tea and mint leaves. Cover the pot and let it steep for about 3-5 minutes.
4. **Strain and Serve:** Remove the tea bags or strain the loose-leaf tea and mint leaves. Pour the tea into mugs or a teapot.
5. **Optional Flavoring:** Add lemon slices and/or honey or stevia for added flavor, if desired.

Green Tea with Fresh Mint Leaves is a soothing and revitalizing beverage, perfect for a heart-healthy diet. Green tea is rich in antioxidants, particularly catechins, which are known to improve heart health by reducing blood pressure and cholesterol levels. Fresh mint leaves add a refreshing twist and can aid digestion while providing additional antioxidants. This low-calorie drink can be enjoyed hot or cold, with optional lemon slices and honey or stevia for added flavor and sweetness. It's an excellent choice for a calming, nutritious boost.

Cinnamon and Clove Warming Tea

Yield: 4 servings | Prep time: 5 minutes | Cook time: 10 minutes

- **4 cups water**
- **2 cinnamon sticks**
- **8 whole cloves**
- **Optional: honey or stevia for sweetness**
- **Optional: lemon slices for garnish**

Nutritional Information:
Approximately 5 calories,
0g protein,
2g carbohydrates,
0g fat,
1g fiber,
0mg cholesterol,
10mg sodium,
15mg potassium.

1. **Boil Water:** In a pot, bring 4 cups of water to a rolling boil.
2. **Add Spices:** Once the water is boiling, add the cinnamon sticks and cloves to the pot.
3. **Simmer:** Lower the heat to medium-low and let the mixture simmer for about 8-10 minutes.
4. **Strain and Serve:** Remove the cinnamon sticks and cloves by straining the liquid. Pour the tea into mugs or a teapot.
5. **Optional Flavoring:** Add honey or stevia and/or lemon slices for additional flavor if desired.

Cinnamon and Clove Warming Tea is a comforting and aromatic drink, ideal for a heart-healthy diet. Cinnamon has been shown to reduce inflammation and lower blood sugar levels, contributing to cardiovascular health. Cloves are rich in antioxidants and have anti-inflammatory properties that support overall heart function. This low-calorie tea is perfect for warming up on a cold day, with the option to add honey or stevia for a touch of sweetness and lemon slices for a citrusy twist. Enjoy this soothing blend to promote heart wellness and relaxation.

Dandelion Root and Burdock Detox Tea

Yield: 4 servings | Prep time: 5 minutes | Cook time: 20 minutes

- **4 cups filtered water**
- **2 tablespoons dried dandelion root**
- **2 tablespoons dried burdock root**
- **Optional: 1-2 teaspoons honey or stevia for sweetness**
- **Optional: lemon slices for garnish**

Nutritional Information:
Approximately 10 calories,
0g protein,
2g carbohydrates,
0g fat,
1g fiber,
0mg cholesterol,
5mg sodium,
20mg potassium.

1. **Boil Water:** In a pot, bring 4 cups of filtered water to a boil.
2. **Add Roots:** Once the water reaches a boil, add the dandelion root and burdock root to the pot.
3. **Simmer:** Lower the heat to medium-low, cover the pot, and let the mixture simmer for about 15-20 minutes.
4. **Strain and Serve:** After simmering, strain the tea to remove the roots. Pour into mugs or a teapot for serving.
5. **Optional Flavoring:** Add honey or stevia for sweetness, and lemon slices for garnish, if desired.

Dandelion Root and Burdock Detox Tea is a powerful blend designed to support liver function and overall detoxification, making it an excellent addition to a heart-healthy diet. Dandelion root is known for its diuretic properties, aiding in flushing out toxins and reducing water retention, which can help manage blood pressure. Burdock root is rich in antioxidants and has anti-inflammatory benefits, contributing to overall cardiovascular health. Enjoy this nourishing tea with optional honey or stevia for sweetness and lemon slices for a refreshing touch.

Lemon Balm and Honey Calming Tea

Yield: 4 servings | **Prep time:** 5 minutes | **Cook time:** 10 minutes

- **4 cups filtered water**
- **2 tablespoons dried lemon balm leaves**
- **1-2 teaspoons honey, optional for sweetness**
- **Optional: Lemon slices for garnish**

1. **Boil Water:** In a pot, bring 4 cups of filtered water to a boil.
2. **Add Lemon Balm:** Once the water reaches a boil, add the dried lemon balm leaves to the pot.
3. **Steep:** Lower the heat to low, cover the pot, and allow the tea to steep for 7-10 minutes.
4. **Strain and Serve:** After steeping, strain the tea to remove the leaves. Pour into mugs or a teapot for serving.
5. **Optional Flavoring:** Add honey for sweetness and lemon slices for garnish, if desired.

Nutritional Information:
Approximately 5 calories,
0g protein,
1g carbohydrates,
0g fat,
0g fiber,
0mg cholesterol,
10mg sodium,
15mg potassium.

Lemon Balm and Honey Calming Tea is a soothing blend perfect for promoting relaxation and reducing stress, which are vital for heart health. Lemon balm is known for its calming effects, helping to lower stress and anxiety, which can positively impact blood pressure and heart rate. The optional addition of honey adds natural sweetness without refined sugars, making it a heart-friendly choice. Enjoy this gentle tea with optional lemon slices for added flavor and a calming ritual in your heart-healthy diet.

Make Your Table Look Beautiful!

Table Setting

Mastering the Art of Table Setting: A Guide to Elegance

Setting a table may seem like a mundane task, but it is an art form that can transform any meal into a memorable dining experience. Whether it's a casual brunch with friends or a formal dinner party, knowing how to properly set a table adds a touch of elegance and sophistication to any occasion. Here's a comprehensive guide to help you master the art of table setting:

1. **Start with a Clean Slate:** Before you begin setting the table, ensure that your tablecloth or placemats are clean and wrinkle-free. A well-prepared surface sets the stage for a polished presentation.

2. **Lay the Foundation:** Begin by placing a dinner plate at the center of each setting. Align it about an inch from the edge of the table. If you're using chargers or placemats, position them beneath the dinner plates for an added layer of elegance.

3. **Arrange the Utensils:** Utensils should be placed in the order they will be used, starting from the outside and working inward. On the left side of the plate, place the dinner fork followed by the salad fork. On the right side, place the dinner knife with the blade facing the plate, then the soup spoon, and finally the dessert spoon or fork horizontally above the plate.

4. **Position the Glassware:** To the right of the dinner plate, arrange the water glass above the knife, followed by the wine or champagne glasses. If serving multiple types of wine, arrange the glasses in the order they will be used, with white wine placed before red wine.

2. **Add the Finishing Touches:** Place the napkin either to the left of the forks or neatly folded on the dinner plate. Alternatively, you can get creative with napkin folding techniques to add a decorative flair. Consider adding a decorative centerpiece, such as fresh flowers or a candle arrangement, to complete the table setting.

3. **Consider Special Touches:** Tailor your table setting to suit the occasion and theme of your event. For formal dinners, use place cards to assign seating and incorporate elegant napkin rings. For more casual gatherings, opt for playful napkin folds and colorful accents.

4. **Maintain Symmetry and Balance:** Ensure that each place setting is evenly spaced and aligned for a visually pleasing presentation. Pay attention to symmetry and balance, keeping the overall look cohesive and harmonious.

5. **Take Pride in Presentation:** Setting the table is not just about functionality; it's about creating an inviting atmosphere and setting the tone for the meal ahead. Take pride in your table setting skills and enjoy the pleasure of hosting guests in style.

Mastering the art of table setting elevates the dining experience and adds a touch of refinement to any occasion. With attention to detail and a creative eye, you can transform even the simplest meal into a memorable feast for the senses.

Conclusion

As we conclude this exploration into the realm of heart-healthy living, let the echo of these pages resonate as a reminder that nourishing your heart extends far beyond dietary choices; it's a holistic journey encompassing mindful nutrition, regular exercise, and a positive mindset. In the symphony of well-being, each note played—the wholesome meals relished, the invigorating exercises embraced, and the optimistic mindset cultivated—composes the melody of a heart in harmony. Remember, this is not a destination but an ongoing voyage, a celebration of progress, not perfection. With heartfelt gratitude for sharing this journey, may your heart continue to beat with vitality, and may your life be a harmonious interplay of health, joy, and resilience.

Appendix 1

Measurement Conversion Chart

Volume: Liquid Conversion

Metric	Imperial	USA
250 ml	8 fl ounce	1 cup
150 ml	5 fl ounce	2/3 cup
120 ml	4 fl ounce	½ cup
75 ml	2 ½ fl ounce	1/3 cup
60 ml	2 fl ounce	¼cup
15 ml	½ fl ounce	1 tablespoon
180 ml	6 fl ounce	3/4 cup

Weight Conversion

½ ounce	15 grams
2 ounce	60 grams
4 ounce	110 grams
5 ounce	140 grams
6 ounce	170 grams
7 ounce	200 grams
8 ounce	225 grams
9 ounce	255 grams
10 ounce	280 grams
11 ounce	310 grams
12 ounce	340 grams
13 ounce	370 grams
14 ounce	400 grams
15 ounce	425 grams
1 pound	450 grams

Spoons

1 tablespoon	1/16 cup
2 tablespoons	1/8 cup
10 tablespoons	2/3 cup
4 tablespoons	¼cup
5 tablespoons	1/3 cup
8 tablespoons	½ cup
12 tablespoons	3/4 cup
16 tablespoons	1 cup

Almond Flour Conversion

USA	Metric	Imperial
1 tablespoon	6 grams	.2 ounces
¼US cup	24 grams	.8 ounces
1/3 US cup	32 grams	1.1 ounces
1/3 US cup	32 grams	1.1 ounces
1/3 US cup	32 grams	1.1 ounces

Butter

USA	Metric	Imperial
1 cup	227 grams	8 ounce
½ cup	113 grams	4 ounce
1/3 cup	75 grams	2.7 ounce
¼cup	57 grams	2 ounce

Index

Made in the USA
Columbia, SC
17 May 2025

58038883R00076